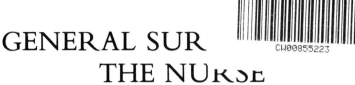

GENERAL SUR
THE NURSE

Robert Horton
MBE, MS, FRCS(ENG)

formerly Consultant Surgeon at the United
Bristol Hospitals

HODDER AND STOUGHTON
LONDON SYDNEY AUCKLAND TORONTO

MODERN NURSING SERIES

General Editors

A. J. HARDING RAINS, MS, FRCS
Regional Dean, British Postgraduate Medical Federation,
formerly Professor of Surgery, Charing Cross Hospital Medical School,
Honorary Consultant Surgeon to the Army

MISS SUSAN E. NORMAN, SRN, NDN cert, RNT
Tutor for Staff Development, The Nightingale School, St. Thomas's Hospital,
London

MRS JEAN HEATH, BA, SRN, SCM, Cert Ed
National Health Service Learning Resources Unit, Sheffield City Polytechnic

This Series caters for the needs of a wide range of nursing, medical and ancillary
professions. A complete list of titles is available from the Publisher.

British Library Cataloguing in Publication Data

Horton, Robert
General surgery and the nurse.—(Modern nursing
series)
1. Surgery
I. Title   II. Series
617.0024613   RT65

ISBN 0 340 33376 6

First published 1983

Typeset in 11/12pt Bembo (Monophoto)
by Macmillan India Ltd, Bangalore

Printed in Great Britain
for Hodder and Stoughton Educational,
a division of Hodder and Stoughton Ltd,
Mill Road, Dunton Green, Sevenoaks, Kent
by Biddles Ltd, Guildford, Surrey

Editors' Foreword

This well established series of books reflects contemporary nursing and health care practice. It is used by a wide range of nursing, medical and ancillary professions and encompasses titles suitable for different levels of experience from those in training to those who have qualified.

Members of the nursing professions need to be highly informed and to keep critically abreast of demanding changes in attitudes and technology. The series therefore continues to grow with new titles being added to the list and existing titles being updated regularly. Its aim is to promote sound understanding by presenting essential facts clearly and concisely. We hope this will lead to nursing care of the highest standard.

Preface

When a patient is admitted to hospital for an operation he is likely to be concerned if not frightened. He is in a strange environment and facing a new and disturbing experience. Although the consultant in charge of the case will have done his best to explain the operation and to allay the patient's fears the nurse will be his nearest friend and prop while he is in hospital.

The object of this book is twofold. First to explain the pre- and postoperative treatment of some of the common operations of general surgery. It also tries to explain the operative procedures and their purpose from the basis of anatomy, physiology, and pathology. I hope this will help nurses to give comfort to their patients as well as giving added interest to the nursing care.

It is a pleasure to acknowledge my thanks to many colleagues both medical and nursing who have given me help and advice. In particular I should like to thank my friend and colleague Professor Harding Rains who has always been a source of encouragement.

The superb drawings are the work of Mr Jack Bridger Chalker, ARCA, RWA, ASIA, a distinguished Bristol and West Country artist and designer and formerly War Artist with the Australian Army in the Far East. His clear drawings are a substantial contribution and I am most grateful to him for the work he has done.

Finally I should like to thank my wife, Pip, for her untiring efforts in typing the script.

Contents

Wounds and their Treatment

Healing by Primary Intention

A clean surgical wound or incision is closed in layers. The surgeon's objective is to bring each layer together so that there is no space in the depth of the wound which will fill with serum and blood and cause delay in healing. The muscle and fascial layer is usually closed with nylon which gives strength to the wound. A variety of techniques is used to close the fat and skin but both must be closed to ensure that there is no space in the fat layer under the skin (Fig. 1, top). Some surgeons close the skin with metal clips which have to be removed with a special clip remover and recently, particularly in the United States, there has been a trend to close the skin with metal staples. These are smaller than clips and cause an insignificant scar, but are expensive.

Such a wound is expected to heal by primary intention. Immediately following suture the small gap between the coapted edges fills with serum and blood. An acute inflammatory reaction begins in the tissue at the edges of the wound and new cells grow out from the edges to meet. In the fat layer these cells are fibroblasts which lay down a substance called collagen which is the basis of a fibrous scar. On the surface, the skin cells grow from each side of the wound to meet and heal the defect. Healing is complete when the injury is fully replaced by living tissue.

Care of a Clean Surgical Wound

Clean surgical wounds generally come from the operating theatre with some sort of cover. This may be a spray which dries to form a thin layer impervious to bacteria. More often some form of dressing is used. Simple gauze adheres to wounds and is not much used. It has been replaced by a variety of non adherent dressings many of which are supplied attached to a plaster which will stick the dressing to the skin. Op-Site (Smith Nephew Ltd) is a transparent dressing which enables the nurses and surgeons to observe progress without removal of the dressing and exposure of the wound to the risk of ward infection. It is generally unwise to take down a dressing until it is time to remove sutures. Suture removal can be done as early as the fourth day if the subcutaneous fat is well sutured and there is no tension on the skin wound. However, if there is tension the sutures should be left much longer, e.g. an incision at the back of the calf should have the sutures in place for ten days. If sutures are left in much longer than ten days they begin to show a red reaction around the suture hole and this may be followed by discomfort and infection.

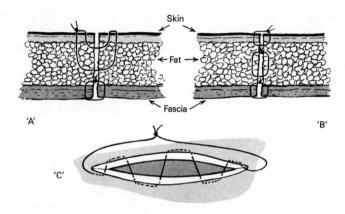

Suture techniques for skin closure
In 'A' and 'B' the fascia is closed with strong nylon
In 'A' the skin and fat are closed with a single suture called a vertical mattress
In 'B' the fat and skin are closed with two separate sutures

'C' shows a suture called a subcuticular suture which passes from side to side and leaves no suture marks along incision

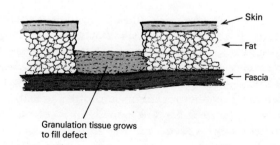

Healing by secondary intention. After defect is filled with granulation tissue the skin grows over the surface

Fig I

Healing by Secondary Intention

Healing by primary intention cannot take place if the edges of the wound are not coapted. This may be because the surgeon has deliberately not closed the wound completely or it may result from infection in a sutured wound which breaks open with separation of the edges. The base of such a wound is usually grey or yellow and this is a thin layer of dead tissue called a slough. The initial treatment is to clean the wound and to await the separation of the slough. Many nurses have their own special preference but Eusol (Edinburgh University solution of lime) has been popular since its introduction in the First World War. To prevent its adhesion to the wound and dressings it is usually used in equal parts with liquid paraffin.

When the slough separates a red, granular surface which bleeds easily is revealed. This is called granulation tissue and it will grow to fill the defect in the wound. At the same time the skin grows in from the edges covering the granulation tissue. The final closure of the wound is assisted by a process of contracture at the base of the wound which reduces the area to be closed. The final result of secondary intention healing is an unsightly scar (Fig. 1, bottom).

If the skin defect is too large for natural closure by growth of skin from the edges the process is completed by the surgeon who does a skin grafting operation.

Management of a Painful Dressing

Some surgeons advise an injection of pethidine about half an hour before doing a dressing which is extensive and likely to be painful.

Another technique is to use a mixture of equal parts of nitrous oxide and oxygen (Entonox) which gives complete relief from pain with safety. The patient is given a mask through which he can inhale the gas mixture. The gas is delivered from a special machine which releases gas in response to a strong inhalation. As the patient continues to breathe he becomes free from pain and also somewhat drowsy. At this stage his hand drops from his face so that inhalation from the mask ceases and the effects of the gas wear off. The patient can use the gas to relieve pain as he wishes.

Complications of Surgical Wounds

The most important and common complications are:

1 **Infection** which is discussed in Chapter 2.

2 **Dihiscence** – this means a complete breakdown of the wound. It sometimes occurs in abdominal incisions and is due to a variety of causes such as poor technique, intestinal distension or infection of the wound.

3 **Keloid** is a complication in which there is an overgrowth of scar tissue resulting in a heaped-up, ugly, scar. It occurs most commonly in Negroes and following the healing of burns. Excision results in a recurrent keloid scar and there is no effective treatment. Fortunately most keloids regress over a period of about two years.

2

Infections and their Treatment

A person has an infection when living organisms enter the body and invade the tissues. Most infections are caused by bacteria but viruses, fungi and larger organisms such as the malaria parasite can also cause illness by entering the tissues.

Most infections seen in surgical practice are caused by bacteria. Bacteria exist everywhere in nature. They are within the body and on the skin. They are present in soil and culture plates left exposed in a room will quickly grow bacteria showing them to be floating in air, possibly on particles of dust. Indeed bacteria are everywhere. Bacteria which are normally present in the body are not harmful. In some cases they do positive good and if the normal bacteria in the colon are eradicated with antibiotics dangerous bacteria and fungi may grow in their place and cause serious bowel infection. Bacteria which are normally present are called commensals. Those which invade the tissues and cause infections are called pathogens or pathogenic bacteria. However, bacteria which are normally present in the colon are only harmless so long as they remain in their natural habitat. Once colon bacteria escape into the tissues they cause a dangerous and spreading infection which may be fatal without treatment.

Bacteria are very small and can only be seen with a powerful microscope. There are many different types of pathogenic bacteria which cause characteristic clinical features of invasiveness. However, all infections cause certain basic responses from the body.

1   Local Response to Infection

Once bacteria invade the tissues there is a local response which is designed to destroy the invading bacteria. Certain cells in the blood called polymorphonuclear leucocytes pass through the capillary walls to surround the bacteria. These cells are also called the white blood cells (WBCs) and they have the ability to ingest foreign invaders such as bacteria. As a result the bacteria are digested in the cell but of course many white cells die in the battle which ensues. In addition plasma leaves the capillaries and floods around the invading bacteria. Plasma contains substances called antibodies which can kill bacteria.

The local effects of an infection are very obvious. There is an increase in blood supply to the part to bring more cells and plasma to repel the infection and this causes the site of infection to be hot and red. The outpouring of plasma causes swelling and the increased pressure resulting from the swelling is painful. These signs of redness, swelling, heat and pain have been known as the cardinal signs of inflammation for nearly 2000 years. Such an area of inflammation is called cellulitis. If the battle is short and there is very little local damage to tissue the inflammation will subside and the part return to normal, a process which is called resolution. In other cases a fierce battle ensues between the body and the invading bacteria during which bacteria and phagocytes die together with some of the local tissue. This dead tissue liquifies to form a collection of pus which is called an abscess. Eventually an abscess makes its way to the surface and discharges but the process is generally shortened by an incision made by the surgeon. At the end of such an acute infection there is much dead tissue to be cleared up and this is done by the phagocytic cells, which are scavengers, clearing up the mess by absorbing dead and dying debris. Once all is clear the defect is invaded by new cells which repair the defect leaving a scar.

2   General Response to Infection

The general response to infection includes a stimulus to the bone marrow to produce more white blood cells and this is reflected in the increased white blood cell count which is called leucocytosis. There is also an increase in antibody production which is delivered to the site of infection through the plasma exudate.

Spread of Infection

While the infection is spreading locally it may also spread much further afield as a result of entry of bacteria into the lymphatic and blood vessels. Spread into the lymphatic vessels may cause lymphangitis which is seen as a red line running up the limb. The bacteria are stopped when they reach the lymph nodes which become tender and enlarged. This is called lymphadenitis and is a common feature of any infection. Reaction in the lymph node is a second line of defence and usually prevents further spread.

Bacteria may also enter the blood stream where they can be identified by taking a sample of blood for culture. A small number of bacteria in the blood is called bacteraemia and is not associated with any symptoms. A heavy infection of the blood stream causes a high temperature with rigors and deterioration of general condition. This is called septicaemia. In some cases of septicaemia the bacteria cause abscesses in various parts of the body. This is called pyaemia.

Staphylococcal Infections

There are several types of staphylococcus but the important one is *Staphylococcus aureas.* Infections with *Staphylococcus aureas* cause abscesses with thick yellow pus. A boil is an infection in a hair follicle and a carbuncle is an infection in the subcutaneous fat, usually at the back of the neck, which discharges through several openings.

In hospital practice the importance of the *Staphylococcus aureus* is that it can be a cause of cross infection in surgical cases. A carrier is a person who carries pathogenic bacteria on the body without any sign of infection. Patients and people working in hospital can carry staphylococci in the anterior nares, which is the hairy part just inside the nostril. It is easy for a nurse or doctor to transfer bacteria from their nose to their fingers and so to a patient.

Streptococcal Infections

Streptococcal infections are less serious than staphylococcal infections. The infection tends to spread locally and by lymphatics and pus formation is not marked. The pus is thin and watery. All streptococci are sensitive to penicillin.

Intestinal Bacteria

The stomach and upper part of the intestine are sterile but bacteria are present in the distal part, particularly the colon and rectum where the bacterial content is very high.

The main colon bacteria are, *Escherichia coli (E. coli)*, *Bacteroides*, *Streptococci* and *Pseudomonas pyocyanea*. All of these bacteria are pathogenic but are harmless commensals so long as they remain within the colon.

The colon bacteria are responsible for intraperitoneal infections which result from perforation of the colon and appendicitis. They are also responsible for infections in the urinary tract which vary greatly in severity.

Pseudomonas pyocyanea is a dangerous infecting bacteria because it is resistant to most antibiotics. It is particularly liable to infect wounds which have been infected with pyogenic (pus forming) bacteria and which have been treated with antibiotics. The infection is easily recognised because of a typical musty smell and green colouration of the wound and dressings.

Wound Infection

Surgical wounds can get infected in the operating theatre or in the ward.

The principle of modern surgery is the aseptic technique in which everything is sterilised before use. Many disposable materials such as syringes and catheters are sterilised with ionising radiation. Theatre air can be contaminated by ward bacteria floating in on dust particles. This is prevented by introducing filtered, bacteria-free air into the theatre suite under such pressure that air passes from the theatre to the passages leading to the rest of the hospital, rather than in the reverse direction.

Dressings, sponges, gowns and instruments are sterilised in an autoclave. This works on the principle of a pressure cooker so that the objects to be sterilised are exposed to steam at 134 °C. Some bacteria, including *Clostridia*, can adopt a spore form which may be compared to animal hibernation. The spore form of a bacteria is much more resistant to destruction. At the temperature reached in an autoclave spores of tetanus and other clostridia are destroyed, but they are not destroyed by boiling. Ordinary bacteria such as staphylococci are killed at a much lower temperature. Disinfection is a term which means that all living organisms except spores are destroyed. Another source of theatre infection is a member of the theatre staff who is a carrier and in any outbreak of infection a nose swab is taken from all theatre staff.

Ward infections can obviously occur in a similar way but it is difficult for bacteria to penetrate the scab which forms on the surface of a wound and deep seated infections are nearly always due to theatre infection. On the other hand a drain site can easily be infected in the ward.

Several techniques are used to reduce ward infection:

1   Wounds are either sprayed with a liquid which gives an impervious cover or are covered with a dressing. Peeping under the dressing is not wise and transparent dressings make this unnecessary. Unless there is some strong indication, a dressing should not be disturbed until the sutures are due to be removed. Early dressing makes unnecessary work and may result in infection.

2   Drains are usually attached to a closed system so that there is no possibility of contamination with ward bacteria. Corrugated drains left in the dressings are being used less because of the risk of infection.

3   When a dressing has to be changed it is best done in a dressing room equipped with positive pressure ventilation just like the operating theatre.

4   Baths are an obvious source of cross infection. Showers are much safer but many patients are not strong enough to take a shower. The bath must be disinfected after use to minimise the risk of cross infection.

5   The dressing is done with sterilised materials and instruments and a no touch technique as much as possible.

Gas Gangrene

This is a very dangerous infection with *Clostridium welchii* and some other *Clostridia*. These bacteria are anaerobic, which means they cannot live in the presence of oxygen. Gas gangrene is a particular clinical state which may result from infection with these bacteria. Often the case is a road accident and there is dead muscle in the limb resulting from injury to the main artery to the part. This provides the anaerobic conditions which are favourable to the *Clostridia*. As the bacteria thrive they produce gas which can be felt in the tissues and which can be seen as bubbles on an X-ray. In addition, bacteria make enzymes which cause putrefaction of the dead muscle. So the wound in such a case stinks with putrefaction and contains obvious gas. There is also a powerful toxin which makes the patient very ill, with rapid pulse and low blood pressure. If the patients's life is to be saved it is necessary to remove all the dead muscle in which the bacteria can multiply and in some cases this can only be achieved by doing a major amputation.

It is important to remember that not all wounds containing gas are the subject of gas gangrene. In some cases gas can be felt in the wound but there is no putrefaction nor severe toxaemia. These are infections with gas-forming organisms. They are not serious and treatment along the usual lines for an infection is adequate.

Tetanus

Tetanus is a disease caused by infection with a bacteria called *Clostridium tetani*. This organism is anaerobic and may grow in a small, penetrating wound such as caused by a rose thorn. The bacteria multiply in the small pocket of dead tissue at the tip of the injury. The actual wound is insignificant but *Clostridium tetani* produces a very powerful toxin which travels to the spinal cord, where it becomes attached to the motor cells causing an increase in muscle tone followed by convulsions. Stiffness in the face and jaw is often an early symptom, hence the popular name of lockjaw. In severe cases the patient's respiratory muscles are in such spasm that breathing is impossible and death from asphyxia follows.

Tetanus can be prevented by prophylactic inoculation with tetanus toxoid. This is best given in childhood and is free from complications. In the event of an injury which might be followed by tetanus, a booster dose of toxoid is given.

If tetanus develops there is no treatment other than support to keep the patient alive until the effects of the toxin wears off. This takes the form of sedation to prevent spasms. In very severe cases with respiratory difficulty it is necessary to paralyse the patient with drugs and to pass a tube into the trachea to give artificial respiration. This is carried out in an intensive care unit.

Principles of Treatment of Infection

1   Rest

Movement causes compression of an inflamed area and spread of infection is encouraged. The part should be kept at rest. An arm is kept in a sling and if the inflammation is in the leg the patient must remain in bed or at least with the leg elevated.

2   Drainage

Surgical drainage is essential as soon as pus has formed.

3   Antibacterial Agents

The whole management of infections has been revolutionised since the introduction of antibacterial agents in Germany in the thirties. The first drugs to be used were chemicals of the sulphonamide group followed by the introduction of antibiotics during the Second World War. An antibiotic is an antibacterial agent made from living organisms. The first antibiotic was penicillin, made and pioneered in England, and its discovery was to have an unparalleled impact on the treatment of infections. Penicillin has a limited bactericidal range and many bacteria are resistant. Later antibiotics were introduced which were of broader spectrum and at the present time few bacteria cannot be controlled. The important principle is to sample the infecting organism with a swab from the wound. In the microbiology laboratory the swab is cultured and the bacterial sensitivity identified. The report to the doctor should contain information on the basis of which he can prescribe the correct antibiotic which will destroy the particular infecting bacteria. Chemotherapy is still used particularly in urinary infections and those caused by the colon bacteria called *Bacteroides.*

3

Tumours and their Treatment

The treatment of tumours occupies a great deal of any surgeon's time. There are a large number of different types which vary greatly in their behaviour and rate of growth.

A tumour consists of a mass of multiplying cells which form a lump in the body or growing from the skin. This mass of cells is said to be autonomous, which means that it is self governing. The cells grow independently and have no useful function in the body. Tumours are classified as benign and malignant.

Benign Tumours

A benign tumour is strictly noninvasive and is surrounded by a capsule which demarcates it from the rest of the body and gives the surgeon a plane of cleavage in which the tumour can be enucleated. The cells of a benign tumour closely resemble those of the host in which it arises, e.g. a lipoma is a tumour of fat cells. When removed it looks like fat and under the microscope it is made of typical fat cells. Benign tumours tend to be small, but some of the largest of all tumours arising in the ovary (benign cystadenoma) and in the wall of the uterus (fibroids) are benign.

Malignant Tumours

The word cancer is used by the public to describe a malignant tumour. It is not often used by doctors as it is a nonspecific term and also carries emotional overtones.

A malignant tumour is characterised by the fact that it is invasive. Normally the cells of the body adhere together, but the cells of a malignant tumour lack this adhesive property and spread away from the main tumour. There are four main ways in which a malignant tumour spreads:

1   Direct Spread

This means that the cells of the tumour invade any adjacent structure, e.g. a malignant tumour of the breast will invade the muscles and ribs of the chest wall on the deep aspect and the skin on the surface. All malignant tumours have this property and surgical excision becomes difficult and sometimes impossible if a tumour has spread beyond the organ in which it arose.

2 Lymphatic Spread

Malignant cells may invade lymph vessels and be transported with the lymph to the nearest lymph node. Some cells are destroyed in the lymph nodes but sooner or later the malignant cells gain a foothold and begin to multiply causing enlargement of the node. This is called a secondary deposit or metastasis.

3 Blood Stream Spread

Malignant cells may also spread into blood vessels. Veins are more commonly invaded because they have thinner walls than arteries. Once cells gain entry into the blood stream there is no limit to the possibility of spread. If the tumour is in the abdomen the cells enter tributaries of the portal vein so that they are carried with the portal blood to the liver, where secondary deposits or metastases develop. In any malignant tumour within the abdomen the surgeon is anxious about the possibility of metastases in the liver which render the patient incurable. Some cells pass through the liver and proceed in the main circulation to the heart, lungs, back to the heart, and then through the main systemic circulation. As a result secondary deposits or metastases are commonly seen in the lungs and in other organs. For some unknown reason some tumours have a tendency to metastasise to bones. These include tumours of the breast, lung, thyroid, and kidney. Secondary deposits are virtually never seen in skeletal muscle, or the heart and spleen. The reason for this is unknown but there must be some factor which destroys cells in these tissues as they must frequently be invaded by malignant tumour cells.

4 Spread across Cavities

Tumour cells may also spread across cavities. Cells from a tumour of the stomach may separate from the main tumour and drift down through the peritoneal cavity until they rest on the ovaries. At this point they gain a foothold and grow to form a large secondary tumour in the ovary. This is called a Krukenburg tumour after the surgeon who described this combination of a primary tumour in the stomach with a secondary tumour in the ovary. Unless it is successfully treated a malignant tumour is inevitably fatal as it spreads far and wide and takes all the nutrition at the expense of the rest of the body.

Basal Cell Tumour

This tumour is unique in its properties and lies between benign and malignant tumours. It arises in the basal layer of the skin and is locally invasive so that it fulfils the main criterion of a malignant tumour. However it never spreads to the lymphatic nodes or by the blood stream.

Epithelial and Connective Tissue Tumours

Tumours are also classified as epithelial or connective. The epithelial tissues include skin and the linings of the internal tubes such as the intestines. The breast is derived from the skin and is considered as an epithelial tissue. The pancreas and gallbladder develop from the intestine and are also epithelial. The rest of the body is connective tissue. In addition to the supporting tissue such as fibrous tissue and fat the bones and muscles are connective tissue.

Benign Epithelial Tumours

A benign tumour arising from the skin is called a papilloma. The lining of the intestine contains glands which produce the digestive ferments and this is called a glandular epithelium. A benign tumour arising from glandular epithelium is called an adenoma.

Malignant Epithelial Tumours

All the malignant tumours of epithelial tissue are called carcinomas. Those which arise from skin are sometimes called squamous carcinoma and those arising from glandular epithelium (intestine, etc.) are called adenocarcinoma. Intestinal carcinomas sometimes produce mucus just like normal intestinal glands. If this is a prominent feature the tumour is called an adenocarcinoma with mucoid or colloid degeneration. The term degeneration is inaccurate as the mucus is simply a secretion from the cells of the tumour.

Benign Connective Tissue Tumours

Benign tumours of connective tissue are named according to the tissue of origin. A lipoma arises from fat cells and an osteoma from bone. A fibroma is a tumour of fibrous tissue and a neurofibroma arises from cells in the nerve fibres.

Malignant Connective Tissue Tumours

Malignant tumours of connective tissue are called sarcomas. According to the tissue of origin they are called fibrosarcoma, osteosarcoma, liposarcoma, etc. Sarcomas spread locally just like carcinomas but their distant spread is mainly through the blood stream. As the cells generally enter the peripheral blood stream they are carried to the lungs where secondary deposits are usually first seen. Secondary deposits in lungs remain asymptomatic until they are very large and patients being followed up after treatment of a sarcoma should have the chest X-rayed at regular intervals.

Lymphoma

The lymphocyte is a small round cell which normally circulates in the blood comprising about 15 to 40 % of the total white cell count. It leaves the blood stream to pass through the lymph nodes and then re-enters the blood stream. Lymphocytes are normally found in the blood, lymph nodes, thymus, liver and spleen. They have the function of producing immune bodies and so assisting the body to repel invasion by viruses or bacteria. The lymphocyte is derived from a cell called a mast cell which is found in the bone marrow. The mast cell divides to pass through various stages on the way to the mature lymphocyte.

Lymphoma are tumours which are derived from mast cells and lymphocytes. The classification of lymphoma is very complicated but tumours included in the lymphomas are, reticulum cell sarcoma, Hodgkin's disease, and lymphoma. The lymphoma are characterised by enlargement of the lymph nodes together with the liver and spleen. In some cases there is a marked increase of lymphocytes in the blood stream.

The only place for surgery in the treatment is excision of a node for histological examination and exploration of the abdomen for staging of the disease to assist the oncologist in planning treatment.

The treatment of lymphoma is by radiotherapy and chemotherapy.

Developmental Tumours

Teratoma

Teratomas usually arise in the ovary or testis where it is thought that a primitive cell begins to multiply and develop without fertilisation. A teratoma is a tumour which consists of many different sorts of tissue indicating its origin from a primitive cell. In the ovary a teratoma is usually benign and forms a cystic tumour which is often given the descriptive name of dermoid cyst. Teratoma of the testis is a malignant, solid tumour.

Embryoma

The embryonic tumours arise from cells which have already specialised to some extent. Embryoma occur in children and the common tumours are nephroblastoma (arising in the kidney), neuroblastoma (arising in the medulla of the adrenal gland), hepatoblastoma (arising in the liver), and medulloblastoma (arising in the medulla of the brain). All these tumours are made from cells of the organ of origin. For example, the nephroblastoma is made up from a mixture of the cells which are present in the kidney while a carcinoma of the kidney arises solely from the cells of the renal tubule.

Embryomas are very malignant.

Hamartoma

The suffix '-oma' means tumour but it is not always a tumour in the sense of a growth or malignant tumour and may be used to indicate any lump. The term haematoma is used to describe a lump of blood in the tissues following trauma. A hamartoma is a malformation which forms a lump. A variety of cells may be present but the important distinction is that it is not a true tumour and does not show any tendency to grow or spread like a tumour. A typical malformation or hamartoma is the haemangioma which is a malformation of blood vessels forming a red lump on a baby's face. Left alone this particular hamartoma disappears spontaneously.

Treatment of Tumours

Patients with malignant tumours are often treated by surgeons in the first place. However, the other aspects of treatment are now carried out by specialists in the field of malignant tumours called oncologists who work in an oncology department. The best interests of patients are often served by surgeon and oncologist working together in combined clinics.

Benign tumours are often left untreated. The indications for surgical removal may be cosmetic. Sometimes a benign tumour interferes with function and is best removed.

Malignant tumours are always treated if at all possible. The primary treatment is usually surgical excision and the operation should be designed to remove the primary tumour and also the possible routes of lymphatic spread. In some tumours such as an osteosarcoma of bone it may be necessary to amputate a limb to achieve the principle of wide excision.

Treatment with radiotherapy is also extensively used either as primary treatment or as an additional safeguard following surgical excision.

Some tumours are hormone dependent. This means that they grow well in a particular hormone environment and it may be possible to inhibit their growth by altering this environment. Carcinoma of the breast and prostate are examples of tumours which can be treated with hormones.

A fourth line of treatment consists of the use of a variety of chemicals which are given orally or by injection. This is called chemotherapy. Chemotherapy has revolutionised the prognosis of some tumours which were almost uniformly fatal. It is used as primary treatment in some cases such as leukaemia and lymphoma and in many other instances when recurrence takes place after primary surgical excision.

The use of chemotherapy or hormones is now being tried following various operations for cancer even if the surgeon believes he has removed the growth completely. This is called adjuvant therapy and is still under trial.

4

General Management of
Surgical Cases

In the management of surgical cases special techniques are used to support the patient and to assist normal physiological functions. These are referred to in the different sections but nurses need a detailed knowledge of the following procedures.

The Gastric Tube

There are a variety of different tubes which can be left in the stomach to aspirate gastric contents. Sometimes these are referred to as Ryle's tubes. John Ryle was a physician who introduced this tube about 50 years ago to investigate gastric function. It is now used for patient care when the surgeon wishes to keep the stomach empty and so to prevent vomiting. Gastric tubes are made of plastic and commonly used sizes vary from about 10 to 16 Fr diameter. The tip is usually radio-opaque so that the position of the end of the tube can be identified by X-ray. Some also have a lead weight in the tip which assists the patient in swallowing the tube but the more rigid tubes do not need a weighted tip. All gastric tubes are supplied sterile from the manufacturers and are marked with a line at about 18 inches (45 cm). When this point reaches the nose the tip should be in the stomach which is 16 inches (40 cm) from the nostril. Some tubes have additional marks. As patients vary in size a rough guide to the length of tube needed to reach the middle of the stomach is the distance from the tip of the nose to the umbilicus. Before passing the tube the whole procedure is explained to the patient and he is screened to ensure privacy. Nasogastric tubes are often passed while the patient is anaesthetised. If he is conscious it is best done with the patient sitting up. The tube is removed from the plastic bag, lubricated with liquid paraffin or KY Jelly and passed through one nostril. No force should be used and if the tube does not pass easily the opposite nostril should be tried. If both nostrils are blocked the tube has to be passed through the mouth. When the tube reaches the back of the nose it strikes the back of the pharynx and turns down. Sometimes it bends forwards and comes into the mouth. If this happens it must be withdrawn and a further attempt made to pass it down into the oesophagus. The patient is asked to swallow and sipping a little water helps the tube to go down. Nurses will be called on to pass a gastric tube in patients who are receiving nonsurgical treatment for intestinal obstruction. Most patients having abdominal surgery will return from theatre with a gastric tube in position but in these cases the tube is passed by the anaesthetist during the operation while the patient is under the anaesthetic.

Management of a Gastric Tube

Once the tube is in position it is taped to the nose or some other convenient and comfortable part with 1 cm Micropore. A 60 ml syringe is attached to the end of the tube and used to aspirate the gastric contents. The aspiration is continued until the stomach is empty and the stomach contents placed in a conical plastic flask so that the amount can be measured and entered on the fluid chart. The tube is connected to a bag which is pinned to the patient's clothes. In some cases the doctor will ask for regular aspiration at prescribed intervals. All aspirate is charted.

Intravenous Infusion

In modern surgery it is often necessary to give fluid intravenously. The fluids include electrolyte solutions in water, blood, blood substitutes, and food such as protein, fat and glucose.

While intravenous infusion may be life saving there are also dangers and very careful adherence to technique is necessary if these dangers are to be avoided.

One of the most dangerous risks is the introduction of infection through an intravenous infusion. The bacteria are introduced directly into the blood stream and the patient suffers from septicaemia. Setting up an intravenous infusion is an operation to be carried out with a strict aseptic technique. Another risk is the introduction of air into the circulation, but modern intravenous sets are supplied with valves which prevent the passage of air into the circulation when the fluid in the bag has all run into the vein. During the transfusion of blood there is a risk of introducing small particles which are called microemboli. If delivered into the vein in large numbers these microemboli, which are delivered to the lung, will obstruct the blood vessels perfusing the lung and interfere with the oxygenation of the blood. An additional filter is placed in the system when blood is being transfused to remove these particles.

Intravenous Fluid Bags (Fig. 2)

Intravenous fluid is now supplied sterile from the manufacturer in plastic bags labelled with the contents. There is a hole at the top of the bag which is used to hang it from a hook on the drip stand. At the other end there are two outlets. One of these can be used to inject additives such as potassium chloride to the contents of the bag. The other is covered with a removable cap which keeps the end sterile. The giving set is attached to the bag after removal of this cap.

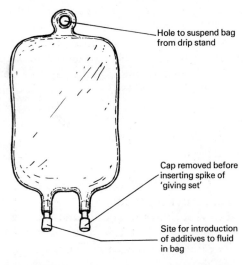

Hole to suspend bag from drip stand

Cap removed before inserting spike of 'giving set'

Site for introduction of additives to fluid in bag

Fig 2   Intravenous fluid bag

The Giving Set (Fig. 3)

This is the part of the apparatus which connects the bag with the cannula or needle. If the giving set is not long enough for the comfort of a mobile patient, an extension $1\frac{1}{4}$ metres in length can be added. The plastic tube above the two chambers on the giving set is covered with a cap to ensure sterility. When this is removed a sharply spiked end is disclosed and this is pushed into the delivery tube from the bag where it breaks a seal within the tube and allows the flow of fluid from the bag. The first chamber on the set is the filtration chamber which is

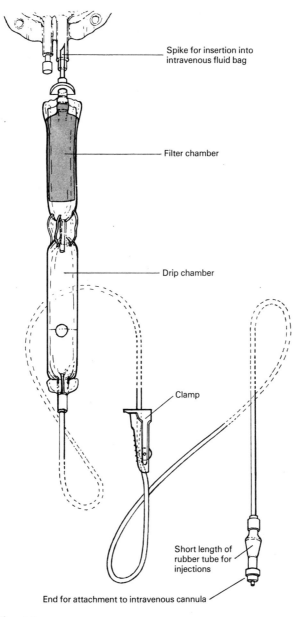

Spike for insertion into
intravenous fluid bag

Filter chamber

Drip chamber

Clamp

Short length of
rubber tube for
injections

End for attachment to intravenous cannula

Fig 3 The giving set

designed to remove any small particles. This can be cleared of air by squeezing which causes the air to rise to the air bubble above the fluid in the bag. The next chamber is the drip chamber which is half filled with air and fluid by squeezing out half the air. The flow can be observed as the fluid drips through the chamber and the rate altered by adjustment of the control. The drip chamber also contains a small floating ball which acts as a ball valve and seals the outlet of the drip chamber when all the fluid from the bag has run into the patient's vein. The plastic tube of the giving set cannot be punctured with a needle but there is a short length of rubber tube at the lower end which can be used for injections. An injection directly into the intravenous line is called a bolus injection and because of the possibility of a serious sensitivity reaction the first bolus injection is always given by a doctor. Subsequent bolus injections may be given by a qualified nurse but this is optional and the nurse's agreement is required.

The Intravenous Cannula (Fig. 4)

There are numerous possible sites for intravenous therapy. Leg veins are best avoided as the patient does not usually move a leg with an intravenous line and this predisposes to vein thrombosis and pulmonary embolism. The doctor will also avoid putting the cannula in front of the elbow joint because bending the elbow may dislodge the cannula.

There are a variety of intravenous cannulae but all depend on the principle that a needle covered with a soft plastic cannula is put into the vein. When blood flows back from the needle showing it to be in

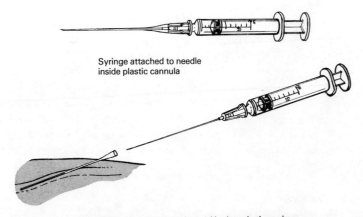

Syringe attached to needle
inside plastic cannula

After the cannula has been located in the vein the syringe
and needle are withdrawn leaving the cannula in the vein .
The intravenous 'giving set' is then attached to the cannula

Fig 4   Intravenous cannula

the vein the needle is removed leaving the soft atraumatic cannula in the vein. The giving set which is already attached to a bag and filled with fluid is then attached to the cannula and the cannula fixed securely to the arm.

Management of an Intravenous Infusion

The doctor assesses the patient's condition daily. This is partly done by clinical observations but often this is aided by sending blood for biochemical examination. The fluid requirements for the next 24 hours are prescribed in writing and it is the responsibility of the nurse to see that the correct volume and type of intravenous fluid is given. Before setting up a new bag of fluid it is carefully examined against the light. It should be perfectly clear and if any floating particles are seen it must be sent back to the pharmacy for examination. The nurse is responsible for seeing that the correct fluid is given to the correct patient and this should be checked by two nurses before being set up. A strict aseptic technique is observed when the bag is changed. If the infusion will not run fast enough or if it stops completely the doctor must be informed. It is more important to infuse the correct volume than to keep the rate constant. If the volume of fluid has fallen behind schedule the rate may be increased to catch up so that by the end of the 24 hour period the fluid prescribed has in fact been given to the patient.

Changing the Giving Set

The DHSS advise the changing of giving sets every 24 hours. The object of this is to reduce the possibility of septicaemia resulting from the growth of bacteria in a giving set. However, this rule is not always followed as it is expensive and many house surgeons believe that frequent changing of the giving set may dislodge the cannula and cause the drip to stop. The giving set must be changed after a blood transfusion and it should be changed daily during intravenous feeding which may block the tubes.

Problems with Intravenous Infusions

The most common difficulty is that the intravenous runs slowly and then stops. This is often due to phlebitis in the vein which is inflamed

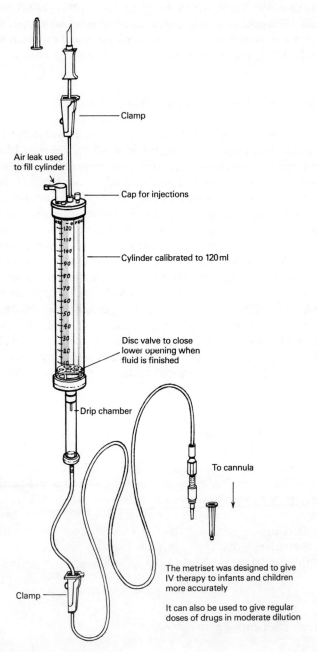

Clamp

Air leak used
to fill cylinder

Cap for injections

Cylinder calibrated to 120 ml

Disc valve to close
lower opening when
fluid is finished

Drip chamber

To cannula

The metriset was designed to give
IV therapy to infants and children
more accurately

It can also be used to give regular
doses of drugs in moderate dilution

Clamp

Fig 5   Metriset

as a result of the fluid which is being infused. The vein becomes red and painful. When this happens the doctor should be informed as the drip site has to be changed even if it is still running. Leakage is another fault which can usually be corrected by tightening a loose fitting.

Introduction of Additives to Intravenous Infusions

Some materials can be added to the bag before it is attached to the giving set. This is done by injecting it through the special plug on the bag (Fig. 2). It is also possible to give an injection of, for example, an antibiotic by putting a needle into the rubber connection which is found just above the cannula end of the giving set. However, the bolus injection of any drug may at times be followed by a severe reaction. A nurse's training is not designed to deal with such an emergency and nurses are not allowed to give a first intravenous injection. To overcome the problem of calling the doctor for all intravenous injections, often in the middle of the night, a 'Metriset'* can be used. This is a special cylinder which contains 120 ml of fluid. Antibiotic or other prescribed drugs can be added to the fluid and given slowly, so avoiding the risk of a dramatic reaction and also enabling the nurse to give the intravenous drug. This technique allows the injection to be given in a dilution of 120 ml and so much more rapidly than in the usual bag of intravenous fluid which contains 1000 ml (Fig. 5).

*Manufactured for Boots by AHS/International.

5

Blood Transfusion

Blood transfusion is a type of tissue transplantation and like all transplantation of tissues there is a problem of compatibility of the donor cells and protein with the cells and protein of the recipient. The solution of this problem is much more advanced than that concerned with the transplantation of organs. Four main blood groups are recognised and these are called A, B, AB and O. These letters refer to different antigens which are located on the red blood corpuscles of an individual person. Antigens are substances which react with substances called antibodies. In a patient of blood group A the red corpuscles contain antigen A but the blood plasma contains antibody which is anti-B. These particular antigens are called agglutins because if blood of group A with A antigen on the corpuscle is transfused into a patient of group B with anti-A antibodies in the plasma, these antibodies react with the foreign protein (antigen) and cause clumping of the transfused cells, which is called agglutination. This is the cause of the transfusion reaction which results from a transfusion of blood which is incompatible. In addition to the ABO groups there is the rhesus factor. Patients may have blood which is rhesus positive or negative and in Caucasian people about 85 % of patients are rhesus positive. Rhesus positive blood can be given to a rhesus positive patient but if rhesus positive blood is given to a rhesus negative patient he will develop antibodies to the rhesus factor and a second transfusion with rhesus positive blood will cause a transfusion reaction.

Table 4.1 illustrates the combinations which occur. About 90 % of Europeans are of blood groups O or A.

Table 4.1   Blood groups showing their antigen and antibody complement

Blood group	Antigen on cell (Agglutinogen)	Antibody in plasma (Agglutinin)
O	None	Anti-A and B
A	A	Anti-B
B	B	Anti-A
AB	AB	—

It will be seen that there is no antigen on the cells of a person of group O and provided he is also rhesus negative this blood may be used on any patient without risk of a transfusion reaction. People of blood group O negative are known as universal donors and blood of this group can be given in an emergency without cross matching of the recipient with the donor blood. Transfusion of O negative blood is only used in this way in emergency cases because of its rarity; only 15% of group O people are Rh negative.

It is not necessary to consider the effect of the antibody in the donor plasma on the antigen in the recipient cells because the transfused plasma is so diluted in the body that it does not have any effect.

Indications for Blood Transfusion

Blood is used in surgical cases to replace blood lost in an emergency haemorrhage. This may be an accident case such as an abdominal or chest injury, or some sudden catastrophe such as a ruptured abdominal aneurysm or bleeding from a peptic ulcer. Blood transfusion is frequently used during major surgery to partly replace blood lost during the operation. It is also used in patients with chronic anaemia who are scheduled for surgery. In cases of chronic anaemia, the patients blood volume is normal and the defect is a shortage of red blood corpuscles so that it is more logical to transfuse a product called 'packed cells' in which some of the plasma has been removed. The blood which is transfused contains the red cells in a smaller volume of plasma. This makes it easier to restore the patients haemoglobin without overloading the circulation with fluid.

Storage and Organisation

Blood is given under a voluntary scheme by a panel of blood donors. The blood is collected at the transfusion centres where it is stored in plastic bags with a mixture known as CPD. The C stands for citrate, which is the anticoagulant used to prevent coagulation of the stored blood, and PD stand for phosphate and dextrose which help to prolong the life of the blood corpuscles. Blood is stored at 4 to 6 °C in a special refrigerator. Blood must never be stored in an ordinary refrigerator as it is damaged below 4 °C and if transfused would cause a serious transfusion reaction. At the transfusion centre the donor blood is grouped. Blood from a patient needing blood transfusion is sent to the transfusion centre where it is grouped and then crossmatched with blood of the same blood group taken from the blood bank. When a suitable bag or unit of blood is found, it is labelled with the patient's name and number and sent to the hospital together with the request form which now has details of the blood which is supplied. Blood is transported from the transfusion centre to its place of need in special insulated boxes which are kept cold by a container of ice which is carried in the box.

Hospital Technique

If several units of blood have been ordered they will be delivered to the ward or operating theatre in a special insulated transport box containing ice. Blood may be kept in this box for 24 hours but after this it must be returned to the refrigerator in the transfusion unit. Single bags of blood which are delivered to the ward must be used at once. While blood transfusion may be life saving, transfusion of blood of the wrong group which is incompatible may be fatal. Many errors have been made in the past and strict adherence to the rules is necessary if mistakes are to be avoided. Before setting up a blood drip the details of the blood and the patient must be checked by two trained nurses. The details to be checked are: the blood group, the transfusion number on the form from the transfusion unit, the patient's name and the patient's hospital registration number. All these must be checked on the unit of blood and also on the patient's notes and identification wristband. The unit of blood carries a sample

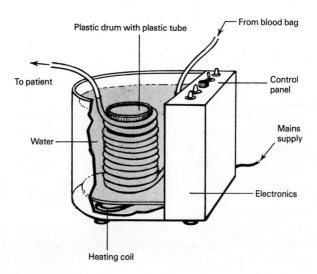

Fig 6 Blood warmer

of the same blood in a small tube attached to the bag. When the blood transfusion is completed the bag is retained in the ward for 24 hours before disposal so that the blood in the attached tube can be re-examined in the laboratory if any adverse transfusion reaction occurs.

If a patient requires a large volume of blood in a short space of time the rapid transfusion of cold blood would result in serious hypothermia. To combat this a blood warmer is used. It is absolutely essential not to warm blood by placing it in hot water as if blood is overheated the red cells break up and a serious transfusion reaction results. The blood warmer is thermostatically controlled and heats the blood to the correct temperature (Fig. 6). Rapid transfusion may also be difficult because the blood will not flow into the collapsed vein fast enough to combat the blood loss. The rate of transfusion can be increased by applying external pressure to the bag.

6

Scientific Aids to Diagnosis

Although the clinical history and examination give the surgeon a good idea of the diagnosis in a particular case the exact diagnosis is often only reached after special and often very sophisticated studies. Exact diagnosis makes for safer surgery and enables the surgeon to plan his operation to give the maximum benefit for the patient. Sometimes the studies show that an operation is unnecessary or that it will not be possible, and then the patient will be saved from an unnecessary exploratory operation. In other cases the tests will indicate some abnormality which needs special preoperative treatment which will make the operation safer for the patient.

All measurements are now recorded in SI units. This is the Système International and is used throughout Europe.

Blood Tests

In collecting blood it is important to know how much is required for an examination and also if the sample is required as clotted blood or as a heparinised specimen which will remain fluid without coagulation. A list of the commonly used tests and the method of collection is contained in the Appendix.

Grouping and Crossmatching

Ten millilitres of blood is collected in a sterile bottle. Usually a request for grouping and cross matching is accompanied by a request for blood for transfusion and a special form completed by the doctor is required.

Full Blood Count

This term is used when the doctor requires a group of tests relative to the cells in the blood. Blood is collected in a bottle containing sequestrene. After placing the blood in the bottle it should be rolled gently between the hands for about a minute to mix the anticoagulant with the blood. Blood consists of two parts, the liquid part or plasma and the cells which are carried round the body in the plasma. There are two types of cell. The red blood corpuscles contain iron and carry oxygen from the lungs to the cells of the body. There is a variation in the number of all cells and chemicals in the blood and the average number of red blood corpuscles is 5 million to a cubic millimetre. The amount of haemoglobin is also estimated and in a normal subject there is about 14.8 grams in 100 millilitres. Patients with a count of haemoglobin below the normal range are anaemic. Those with a level higher than normal are suffering from polycythaemia. Cell counts used to be done laboriously by actually counting but they are now done automatically by a machine. The doctor in the haematology laboratory (the haematologist) looks at a thin smear of blood with a microscope and reports on the appearance of the cells. If the red corpuscles have the normal colour they are said to be normochromic. If they are the normal size they are normocytic. Small cells are called microcytic and large cells are macrocytic. A deficiency of vitamin B12 or folic acid results in the production of macrocytes (large red blood corpuscles) and this can also be studied by estimating the blood level of vitamin B12 and folic acid. An anaemia in which the cells are smaller than normal is a microcytic anaemia and is generally due to a deficiency of iron. This may be a dietary deficiency but it may also be due to a continuous blood loss from a cancer in the stomach or intestine and surgeons are always alerted to the possibility of a serious underlying cause of an iron deficiency or microcytic anaemia.

The other cells in the blood are the white blood cells and the platelets. Platelets are concerned with coagulation and the average number is 250 000 in a millilitre. There are a variety of white blood cells but surgeons are mostly concerned with polymorphonuclear leucocytes (many shaped nucleus white cell). The normal range is between 5000 and 10 000 per millilitre and the number is raised in infections as these cells are part of the response to infection by bacteria.

Erythrocyte Sedimentation Rate (ESR)

In a column of anticoagulated blood the red corpuscles fall or sediment to the bottom of the tube because of the effect of gravity. The normal rate of sedimentation is from 2–10 mm in an hour. In any infection there is an increase in the blood fibrinogen and globulins. This causes the blood corpuscles to clump together so increasing the weight of individual particles and increasing the rate of sedimentation. The sedimentation rate is also increased in cancer. In doubtful cases the ESR can be used to assist the surgeon in making up his mind. A normal ESR suggests that there is neither severe infection nor cancer.

Liver Function Tests

Ten millilitres of blood are collected and placed in a sterile tube for despatch to the biochemistry laboratory. A number of tests are done and reported together. Liver function tests are often used to distinguish between different types of jaundice and they are also used in cases of enlarged liver (hepatomegaly) in which the cause is uncertain. Often the tests are helpful in deciding if an enlarged liver is due to cirrhosis or secondary deposits of cancer.

Blood bilirubin is raised in jaundice and serial estimations show if the jaundice is deepening or fading. The alkaline phosphatase is raised in obstructive jaundice. It is also considerably raised when there are secondary deposits of cancer in the liver even when the patient is not jaundiced. The proteins albumin and globulin are measured in routine liver function tests. Albumin is made in the liver and in liver disease the level of albumin is often low. Some globulin is also made in the liver and in liver disease such as chronic hepatitis and cirrhosis there is increased production of globulin. The blood level of albumin is normally about double that of globulin but in cirrhosis the ratio may be reversed. Certain enzymes normally produced in the liver cells are produced in excess when there is liver cell damage. One such enzyme which is often estimated in liver function tests is the aspartate aminotransferase.

Blood Electrolytes

Five millilitres of blood are collected in a heparin bottle. The level of electrolytes in the blood is normally at a constant level. The most common cause of abnormality in surgical practice is interference with normal absorbtion as a result of interference with intestinal function following abdominal surgery. Certain tumours of the endocrine glands also have dramatic effects on the blood electrolytes. Abnormalities of the blood electrolytes following surgery are corrected with intravenous therapy in which water and electrolytes are given. The amount of water, sodium, chloride and potassium which is needed each day can be calculated by study of the results of the blood electrolytes performed on the previous day. In an emergency case such as intestinal obstruction, the electrolytes can be estimated urgently and intravenous therapy given to correct the abnormality. The risk of the operation is considerably reduced when the blood electrolytes are restored to normal.

The electrolytes which are usually studied are: sodium, chloride, potassium and bicarbonate.

Radioisotope Studies

Electromagnetic radiation varies from very low frequency radio waves through visible light to X-rays and gamma rays to cosmic radiation at the highest frequency.

An atom is a particle consisting of a nucleus surrounded by electrons which are orbiting the nucleus. The nucleus consists of neutrons which are electrically neutral and protons which have a positive charge equal and opposite to that of the orbiting negatively charged electrons. The chemical characteristics of any particular atom are determined by the number of protons. An isotope is an atom with a different number of neutrons in the nucleus. This cannot alter the chemical properties which are determined by the number of protons but the atom is rendered electrically unstable so that it emits alpha and beta particles or gamma rays or a combination of these. Alpha particles penetrate only 1 mm of human tissue and beta particles only 1 cm and therefore isotopes which emit alpha and beta particles are unsuitable for clinical investigation. Gamma rays have great powers of penetration and an isotope which is emitting gamma rays from a deeply placed organ can be identified with a gamma scanner. The half-life of an isotope is the length of time in which its activity decays by half.

The ideal isotope for clinical use should emit gamma rays and should have a short half-life. It should retain its radioactivity long enough for completion of the study but it must not remain in the body emitting radiation long after completion of the test.

Isotopes are made at the Radio Chemical Laboratory at Amersham, England and distributed on request. Radioactive technetium, which is a commonly used isotope in clinical study, has a half-life of only six hours. It is more convenient to deliver radioactive molybdenum which can be converted to the radioactive form of technetium in the local department of medical physics. Technetium can be attached to other chemicals and the particular attachment is determined by the organ which is the subject of study. There is obviously a theoretical risk in handling isotopes. They are transported in a flask surrounded by lead which prevents the passage of gamma rays. The important safety considerations are the time of exposure and the distance from the source. Bearing these facts in mind, when the doctor comes to make the injection he keeps as far as possible from the isotope and gives the injection as quickly as possible. The exposure of the doctor is negligible and even the patient who holds the isotope in the body for some hours receives a minute dose.

Liver Scan

In this study the technetium is attached to colloidal sulphur. A colloid is a preparation which is in the form of very fine particles which are removed from the blood stream by cells of the reticuloendothelial system. These cells have the function of removing any particles and are particularly useful for removal of bacteria. Most reticuloendo-thelial cells are found in the liver and if the liver is scanned 15 minutes after an intravenous injection of colloidal sulphur labelled with technetium, a picture or scan of the liver is obtained. If any large part of the liver is occupied by some other cells, such as a secondary deposit of cancer, then this area does not pick up the isotope and appears as an empty area on the scan. Using this technique a metastasis or other lesion larger than 2 cm can be identified. Scanning, however, cannot tell if the object in the liver is a solid secondary deposit or an innocent cyst.

Bone Scans

Technetium labelled phosphate compounds are used for scanning bone. The bones are scanned four hours after an intravenous injection. An increased uptake shown on the scan indicates that there is increased bone activity. This is a nonspecific finding and may be due to a number of causes. A bone scan may be done as a routine screening test in a patient with known breast cancer but nothing to suggest metastases. It is also done in cases of breast cancer when the patient is complaining of bone pains which might due to secondary deposits. Active arthritis also gives a positive scan and if there is undue activity it is usual to advise an X-ray of the area which is under suspicion.

Thyroid Scans

The thyroid gland is particularly suitable for scanning as it selectively takes iodine from the blood stream. ^{131}Iodine is a suitable isotope with a short half-life which is removed from the blood stream by the cells of the thyroid gland just like other forms of iodine. In this study the isotope is given orally and the thyroid is scanned 24 to 48 hours later. Using this technique it is possible to identify areas with no uptake of iodine and also areas of increased uptake. A colloid cyst or a cancer of the thyroid will not take up iodine and these areas are known as 'cold' nodules. A hyperactive nodule is a rare cause of the disease known as thyrotoxicosis. When there is increased activity in a nodule it is called a 'hot' nodule. Cold nodules are much more frequently seen than hot nodules.

Ultrasound Studies

Sound travels as a mechanical wave form quite different from the electromagnetic waves of visible light and X-rays. The human ear can detect sound when the frequency of the waves lies between 20 and 20 000 hertz (Hz). Sound waves of higher frequency are called ultrasound and these waves are now used in diagnosis. A particular advantage of ultrasonic diagnosis is that the technique is entirely non-invasive. This means that nothing is injected or swallowed. The patient simply lies on a couch and the doctor passes a probe, which is the source of the ultrasonic waves, over the part which is being investigated.

The principle of ultrasonic diagnosis is that when the waves strike an interface in the body some of the sound waves are reflected. These reflections are called echoes. When sound waves are passed through a liver containing secondary deposits of cancer some waves will be reflected at the interfaces between normal liver and cancer deposits and these echoes can be detected by a sensitive receiver. This is generally easier than isotope scanning. A particular advantage of the ultrasound scan is that it is possible to say if a particular object picked up by the scan is solid or cystic. This is not possible with isotope scanning.

Ultrasonic scanning now has very wide range of use and its place in diagnosis is constantly increasing. It is used in obstetrics to diagnose early pregnancy, to detect some foetal abnormalities and in the investigation of the heart. In the field of urology it can be used to distinguish between a cancer of the kidney and a simple cyst which does not require treatment.

Endoscopy

Endoscopy simply means looking inside the body. An instrument called a proctoscope has been used for many years to look inside the rectum and a sigmoidoscope is a straight steel instrument which can be passed for a distance of up to 30 cm so enabling the surgeon to look inside the whole rectum and some of the sigmoid colon. These and other instruments used for endoscopy are rigid and difficult to pass. They are still extensively used especially in Outpatients but a new impetus and importance has been given to endoscopy in recent years because of the development of fibrelight and fibreoptics.

In fibrelight a strong source of light is transmitted to the endoscope through a cable of very small glass fibres. Light travels in straight lines along each individual fibre of glass and when the cable of fibres is bent the light is reflected from the outer circumference of the fibre so keeping inside the fibre and giving a light at the endoscope which is virtually as strong as that in the light source. The advantage of this technique is that a much stronger light is available for the surgeon doing an endoscopy. When the old type rigid sigmoidoscope is used, fibrelight illumination gives much better light than the small electric bulb which was previously used. It is essential to remember that the cable is made from a great many fine glass fibres and that it can be ruined by rough handling or by being dropped on the floor, so fracturing the glass fibres.

A second and more complicated development is fibreoptics. A similar principle is used but the bundle of fibres is so constructed that they are in precisely the same position relative to one another at each end of the cable. This construction is called a coherent bundle and gives a clear and undistorted view to an observer. In the cable that is used for the transmission of light, the fibres are arranged randomly. The advantage of the coherent bundle of fibres is that it can be used to get a clear view and also that the endoscope consisting of fibres of glass can be bent without damaging the view. This is the principle of the fibreoptic endoscopes which can be passed much more easily and safely than the old rigid endoscopes. The fibreoptic cable is difficult and very expensive to manufacture and like the fibrelight cable easily damaged by rough handling.

Fibreoptic endoscopy is a large and rapidly enlarging field of investigation which yields a great deal of information. Two commonly used endoscopies are gastroduodenoscopy and colonoscopy.

Colonoscopy

The colonoscope is 160 cm in length and can be used to examine the whole colon to the caecum. The flexible sigmoidoscope is shorter and of more practical value. Its length is 100 cm and it can be used to examine the colon as far as the splenic flexure.

Colonoscopy does not replace barium enema examination of the rectum and colon which is a well established and safe technique for diagnosis of carcinoma of the colon. Colonoscopy is indicated when the X-ray shows a doubtful shadow which might be a polyp. Colonoscopy can be used to confirm the presence of a polyp and it can also be used to take small pieces for biopsy examination. By using a wire snare the colonoscope can also be used to remove small polyps so saving the patient the risk of a major operation (Fig. 7).

Colonoscopy is often performed in cases of undiagnosed rectal bleeding when a small cancer, polyp, or other lesion may be found which did not show on the barium enema X-ray.

The colon is prepared in one of the ways described in the section on colon surgery and the examination is done with the patient in the left lateral position. No sedation is necessary. The tip of the colonoscope can be bent to negotiate the instrument round the bends of the colon. There are a number of control buttons on the instrument. The colon can be inflated with air and suction may be used to remove fluid obscuring the view. A water jet cleans the glass end of the fibrescope. There is an opening through which a snare can be passed. This is a wire loop which can be used to encircle the stalk of a polyp. As the wire is pulled tight a diathermy current is used so that the polyp is snared off without bleeding. This channel in the endoscope can also be used to take small biopsy specimens.

The colon normally contains methane which is an explosive gas when mixed with oxygen. As a safety precaution the colon is filled with the inert gas carbon dioxide during diathermy operations which might cause a spark and consequently an explosion.

Gastroduodenoscopy

Examination of the stomach and duodenum can be done as an outpatient procedure. The patient must be starved from the previous

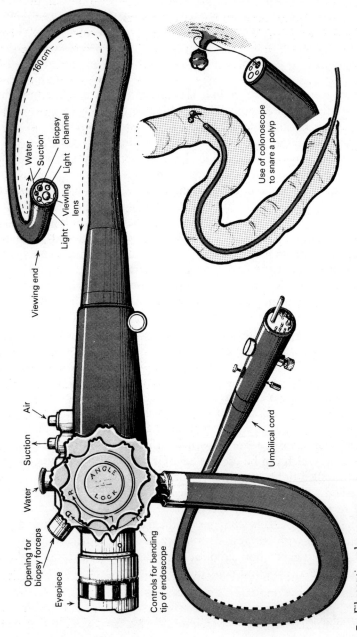

Water
Suction
Biopsy channel
Light
Light
Viewing lens
Viewing end

160cm

Use of colonoscope to snare a polyp

Air
Suction
Water
Opening for biopsy forceps
Eyepiece
ANGLE LOCK
Controls for bending tip of endoscope
Umbilical cord

Fig 7 Fibreoptic colonoscope

night as it is impossible to examine the stomach when it contains food.

The instrument does not differ in principle from the colonoscope which has already been described but passage of the instrument is more trying for the patient. The gastroduodenoscope is 100 cm in length. Surgeons do not all ask for the same premedication but a 30 mg amethocaine lozenge is often given to the patient to suck followed by a 4% lignocaine throat spray to reduce the gagging reflex which the patient feels as the instrument is passed. Some endoscopists try to dispense with any sedation but others use diazepam intravenously just before passing the gastroscope. As soon as it reaches the oesophagus a dental guard is passed over the endoscope so that the patient cannot bite it so fracturing and causing serious damage to the glass fibres.

It is possible to see and biopsy lesions of the oesophagus, stomach and duodenum. One particular advantage over a barium meal examination is the ability to biopsy an ulcer of the stomach which cannot be certainly diagnosed as benign or malignant by X-ray.

Cannulation of the Common Bile Duct

This examination is called endoscopic retrograde cannulation of the common bile and pancreatic ducts (ERCP). It is performed in difficult cases of jaundice when the surgeon has not succeeded in getting a precise diagnosis by other investigations. The examination is similar to gastroduodenoscopy but a special endoscope with a side viewing optical system is used. A fine plastic catheter is passed through a channel in the endoscope and guided through the bile duct papilla into the bile duct. Radio-opaque contrast medium is injected and X-ray films taken to show the bile duct and any abnormality which may be present.

Care of Patients after Gastroduodenoscopy

While the throat is anaesthetised the normal swallowing reflex is abolished because the patient cannot feel food or drink in the back of the throat. Anything taken by mouth during the time that the throat is anaesthetised may go into the trachea with disastrous results. All food and drink must be withheld for at least four hours. If diazepam has been used the patient must be warned that its effect may last for 48 hours and he must not drive a car for this time.

The Servicing of Endoscopes

Although there are very few examples of the transfer of infection attributable to the use of an endoscope it is an obvious possibility. An infection such as dysentery can be transferred by the use of a colonoscope. Pseudomonas is an organism which is inclined to colonise and live in endoscopes and this can cause infection in the bile ducts or intestine if introduced on an endoscope. There is no record of the transfer of hepatitis by endoscopy but it is a theoretical possibility.

Fibreoptic endoscopes cannot be sterilised. Boiling or sterilising in an autoclave will result in total destruction. Thorough cleaning of the outside of the instrument and flushing of the internal channels is of primary importance and makes disinfection more effective. After cleaning with water and detergent the instrument is placed in a disinfectant solution and the internal channels of the fibrescope filled with disinfectant. After ten minutes the whole instrument is washed again to remove all traces of disinfectant. The most effective disinfectant solution is gluteraldehyde but some people show skin sensitivity to gluteraldehyde and technicians should wear gloves. A machine is now available which washes the outside of the endoscope and the internal channels. It operates like a washing machine giving a water wash followed by a wash with gluteraldehyde and a final rinse with water.

Computerised Tomography

The so called CT scan is a highly complicated technological achievement. In very simple terms the body is scanned by X-rays and the scans are analysed and converted into transverse sections by a computer. Computerised tomography was first used for examination of the brain and this is still a most important use. In the brain the CT scan can be used to identify a brain haemorrhage or tumour. In the body the technique produces accurate transverse sections of the trunk. The normal anatomy is clearly shown and any abnormal anatomy or tumour can be seen.

The examination has the great advantage that it is non-invasive. This means that nothing is given to the patient either by mouth or by injection so that he is not disturbed at all and the examination is entirely without risk.

7

Shock

Shock is a clinical condition which is caused by a reduction of blood flow. This results in a reduced flow in the capillaries where oxygen and nutrition is transferred from the blood to the cells. This is called reduced tissue perfusion and is the basic fault in all forms of shock.

There are three main causes of shock:

1 Cardiac Shock

In cardiac shock the reduced tissue perfusion results from sudden partial failure of the heart which is the pump in the system. Often the cause is cardiac ischaemia. Treatment of cardiac shock is outside the scope of this book but it is obvious that the treatment consists of measures to restore effective pumping power in the heart. Another important cause of interference with the pumping action of the heart is a large pulmonary embolus. A pulmonary embolus is a clot of blood which has formed in the leg. If it becomes detached from the vein in which it formed it is swept up into and through the right side of the heart. A large embolus partly obstructs the outflow from the heart and reduces the circulation of the blood.

2 Hypovolaemic Shock

This term simply means that the shock and reduced tissue perfusion results from some condition in which there is not enough fluid in the blood vessels to achieve an effective circulation. The pump is normal but there is not enough blood for it to be effective. There are several important causes of hypovolaemic shock.

The most obvious cause is haemorrhage. There may be external bleeding resulting from an accident or internal in which the blood is lost from the blood vessels but remains within the body. Some examples of this are ruptured spleen in which the blood flows into the peritoneal cavity or a ruptured aneurysm of the aorta in which a large volume of blood leaks from the aorta and forms a retroperitoneal haematoma. Fractures of the large bones such as the femur cause shock in the same way by causing a haematoma in the thigh.

Extensive burns cause shock because the exudate of fluid containing protein from the burn site comes directly from the capillaries. The blood volume is reduced by loss of the plasma. The cellular part of the blood, particularly the red blood corpuscles, are more concentrated and as the loss of plasma continues the haemoglobin rises.

In some other cases shock may result from the loss of fluid and electrolytes which are to some extent replaced from the circulating blood. These cases include acute intestinal obstruction where fluid is lost into the intestine, vomiting, and acute peritonitis where fluid is lost into the intestines and into the peritoneal cavity.

3   Bacteraemic Shock

Certain serious diseases of the colon and urinary tract may be complicated by a special form of septicaemia caused by the bacteria which normally live in the colon and often infect the urinary tract. The most common infection is with *E. coli* which contains a toxin called an endotoxin. If a patient gets a septicaemia with *E. coli* the dead bacteria in the circulation release endotoxin which causes generalised vasodilatation. In this case the state of shock results with a normal heart and normal quantity of circulating blood but the fault lies in the fact that the circulation has become too large to be filled by the amount of blood available and this results in reduced tissue perfusion.

This form of shock is also called endotoxic shock or Gram negative bacterial shock because of the Gram negative staining characteristic of *E. coli*.

Physiology of Shock

Whatever the cause of shock the physiological consequences are the same. As the circulation becomes less effective the blood pressure falls. There are sensors in the aorta and in the carotid artery which pick up this fall in blood pressure and nerve impulses go from the sensors to the brain. In response to nerve impulses reporting a fall in blood pressure the brain sends out messages through the sympathetic nervous system which have a variety of effects. In the skin the result is constriction of the blood vessels (vasoconstriction). As the normal colour of the skin is due to the blood circulating in it this vasoconstriction results in the clinical sign of pallor. The skin is pale in shock because of vasoconstriction and not because of blood loss. As the sympathetic nerves also supply the sweat glands an incidental symptom is excessive sweating.

Sympathetic stimulation of the adrenal gland results in the secretion of adrenalin which causes an increase in the heart rate. There is also vasoconstriction in the viscera and this narrowing of the blood vessels together with acceleration of the heart rate tends to raise the blood pressure.

As the vasoconstriction continues small vessels which are called shunts open up (Fig. 8). These shunts are normally closed but with vasoconstriction they open and allow a circulation to take place. Although this has some advantages the prolonged constriction of the very small vessels causes severe tissue anoxia, i.e. the blood does not reach the tissues which are starved of oxygen. In the kidney this tissue anoxia causes renal function to be depressed and urinary output is reduced and may even stop altogether in a severe case. Another effect is metabolic acidosis. The cells of the body are still living and producing the end-products of life which are normally removed by the blood stream. During the intense vasoconstriction the end products, which are called metabolites because they are the result of metabolism, accumulate in the tissues and small blood vessels. These end products are acid and include lactic acid, and when the vasoconstriction is relieved the acids flood into the circulation causing acidosis. Acidosis is dangerous as it interferes with vital life functions. It also causes vasodilatation and contributes to a further fall in the blood pressure.

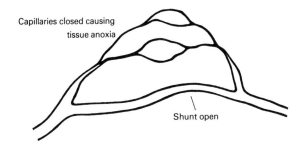

Capillaries closed causing tissue anoxia

Shunt open

Fig 8 Vasoconstriction with open shunt in shock

Management of a Patient with Shock

There are many causes of shock and each case needs treating according to the cause. The physiology is complicated and it is necessary to measure the vital functions at regular intervals to assess the patient's condition and also to prescribe further treatment accurately.

Blood pressure and pulse rate are simple clinical indicators of the patient's condition and should be taken at least every 15 minutes. A falling blood pressure and rising pulse indicate that the shock is increasing.

In serious cases a central venous catheter is used to measure the central venous pressure (CVP). A special catheter is passed into the superior vena cava. There are several routes but a popular technique is to insert the catheter into the subclavian vein where it passes just underneath the clavicle. The catheter is kept open by running a slow infusion of isotonic fluid but it is not used for the main intravenous treatment as this has a small risk of infection in the catheter which can spread to the blood stream. The central venous pressure can be measured as often as indicated and should be within the range of 3 – 10 cm of water with zero at the mid axillary level. Generally a low CVP indicates that the condition has not been adequately treated. Higher than normal levels indicate cardiac failure, possibly the result of overtransfusion.

8

Breast

Anatomy (Fig. 9)

The breast is situated in the fat covering the 2nd to the 6th ribs. There is no capsule but it is loosely attached to the skin and to the underlying chest (pectoral) muscles. The axilla or armpit is bounded by two muscular folds which are called the anterior and posterior folds of the axilla. The breast is somewhat pear shaped and the tail of the breast extends up to the anterior fold and then curves behind it into the axilla. This part of the breast is called the axillary tail.

The breast is a vascular organ with many arteries and veins.

The lymphatic drainage of the breast has particular importance in understanding the spread of breast cancer by this route. Most of the breast drains into lymphatic vessels which pass towards the axilla and enter lymphatic nodes in the axilla. After passing through these nodes

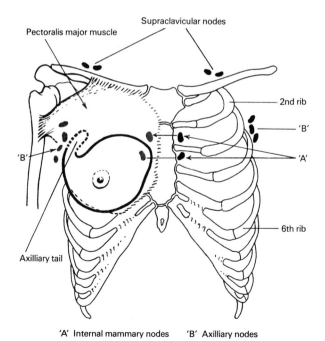

Fig 9 Lymph drainage of breast

the lymph proceeds through lymph vessels which pass through the apex of the axilla and underneath the clavicle (collar bone) to the supraclavicular nodes and thence into the great veins in the neck. Any cancer cells spreading by this route may be held up in any of these nodes where they will multiply causing enlargement of the node and eventually finish in the blood stream to be disseminated all over the body. The medial half of the breast drains into vessels which pass through the spaces between the ribs near the sternum to join nodes which are within the chest and placed alongside an artery called the internal mammary artery. Because of this anatomical relationship these glands are called the internal mammary nodes. The internal mammary artery gives branches which pass through the intercostal spaces to bring blood to the breast.

Physiology

The breast is rudimentary until puberty when it develops. Throughout active sexual life the breast undergoes cyclical changes as a result of a complicated sequence of changes in the secretion of hormones. The breast enlarges and undergoes a varying amount of nodularity during the second half of the cycle and may even develop lumps which the patient can feel. With the onset of menstruation the breast quickly subsides and the tension and nodularity disappear.

Breast Cancer

Cancer is by far the most important disease in the breast and causes about 10 000 deaths in Britain every year. A cancer usually presents to the patient as a painless lump which is found accidentally, often during bathing. Like all malignant tumours a breast cancer spreads locally, by the lymphatic vessels and by the blood vessels. Local spread to the underlying muscle can be detected by the doctor as the lump becomes fixed to the muscle. Attachment to skin causes dimpling of the skin and attachment to the breast ducts causes retraction of the nipple. Some women go to the doctor because of an obvious change in the shape of the breast or nipple. Breast cancer is thought to arise from a single cell which becomes malignant and the cancer grows by repeated division of this original cell until a lump is formed which is large enough for the patient to be able to feel. It is estimated that this may take up to three years and during this time some cells may break off and spread through blood vessels to form micrometastases in bones or other organs. This depressing observation accounts for the fact that some apparently early cases already have distant metastases and others develop them within a year of primary treatment. The most common site of secondary deposits which have been carried by the blood stream is bone – particularly the spine and pelvis. At a later stage they are seen in many other organs including the lungs, liver, brain and skin. The third route for spread of breast cancer is via the lymphatic vessels. Such spread causes enlargement of the lymph nodes in the axilla or in the internal mammary nodes. The axillary nodes are easily felt by the surgeon but those inside the chest cannot be diagnosed.

Breast Screening

Because of the serious nature of the disease and the fact that patients have a better chance of cure if the disease is detected and diagnosed at an early stage, attempts have been made to screen all women. There are two popular techniques at present. The easiest is self examination in which the woman is taught to examine her breast once a month and to report any lump which is persistent. Lumps which vary in size are not malignant. The examination is made at the end of menstruation when breast lumps caused by fibroadenosis (mastitis) are unlikely to cause confusion. Women's magazines and the mass media often campaign on this subject. The second technique is by radiography. This examination, which is called mammography, takes some time and it is logistically impossible to X-ray all women over 35 years old every year. However, there is no doubt that this technique can pick up some early cancers and it may be that women who are particularly at risk should be X-rayed annually.

Diagnosis

Nowadays no surgeon would be prepared to do a mastectomy on clinical evidence alone. When breast cancer is suspected further studies are made to attempt to confirm the diagnosis in the outpatient department.

   1   **Mammography.** This is not absolutely diagnostic but the shadow of a carcinoma is characteristic and fine stippled calcification within this shadow is usually seen.

2 Aspiration Cytology (Fig. 10). This test is done by introducing a 21 FG needle on a 20 ml syringe. Once the needle is in the tumour, maximum suction is applied by withdrawing the plunger of the syringe as much as possible. With this suction maintained the needle is passed through the tumour two or three times and then withdrawn. Although the syringe appears empty it is possible to blow a little fluid from the needle onto a microscope slide. This is left to dry and after suitable staining can be examined for malignant cells.

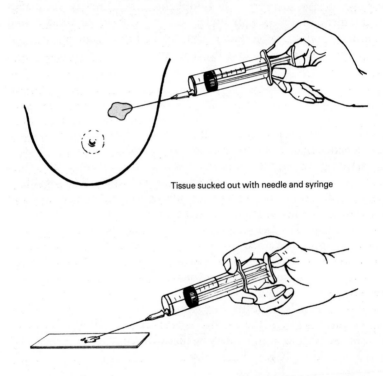

Tissue sucked out with needle and syringe

Material squirted out on to glass slide for microscopic examination

Fig 10 Aspiration cytology

3 Needle Biopsy. Cytology does not require an anaesthetic but 1–2 ml of 1 % lignocaine are needed for needle biopsy. A small nick is made with a scalpel in the anaesthetised skin and the 'Trucut' needle can then be passed into the tumour and a biopsy taken. This small fragment is placed in formal saline and sent to the histology department.

Using these techniques a firm diagnosis can usually be made and the diagnosis and treatment can be discussed with the patient at a second outpatient consultation.

Distant Metastases

At the time of the first consultation it is important to know the stage of the disease. There are a number of staging methods but the one in most common use is the International Staging or TNM in which 'T' stands for tumour, 'N' for lymph nodes, and 'M' for distant metastases. A figure (0, 1 or 2), goes after each letter to represent the extent of the disease locally, in the nodes and in distant organs. The extent of local disease and node involvement is determined by clinical examination. Other investigations are needed to study the organs and their involvement. The chest is X-rayed as a routine to exclude lung metastases. Bone and liver metastases can be studied by scanning after giving the patient a radioactive isotope. These techniques are described in Chapter 6. Scanning may give false positive results especially in bones but any suspicious area seen on the scan is further studied with radiographs. Liver metastases need to be more than 2 cm in diameter to show with this technique.

By using these scanning techniques it is possible to evaluate the stage and extent of the disease, but not all surgeons employ them routinely. Surgical treatment is generally used for patients with what is called early breast cancer. These are the cases in which the disease is confined to the breast and axillary lymph nodes.

After confirmation of the diagnosis the surgeon will give the patient a further consultation to discuss the treatment which is required. At this consultation it is very helpful if the patient's husband is present so that both parties know exactly the surgeon's recommendation.

Surgical Treatment of Early Breast Cancer

There is at the present time no uniform surgical opinion as to the correct primary surgical treatment of breast cancer. A number of different operations will be described and any of these may be seen in different centres of surgery. The first determined attempt to treat breast cancer was by Halstead, who introduced the operation of radical mastectomy in Baltimore in 1894. It is surprising that this very disfiguring operation was done throughout the USA and Great

Britain until the end of the last war. There has been no significant advance in the cure of breast cancer but since 1946 there has been a trend towards lesser operations which are less unacceptable cosmetically without increasing the risk of recurrence.

If a pathological diagnosis has not been made the mastectomy may be preceded by an excision of the lump which is examined by a special technique often called 'frozen section'. The report usually reaches the surgeon within 30 minutes and if positive he can proceed to mastectomy.

Radical Mastectomy

This is the operation originally described by Halstead. The breast is removed together with the main muscles in front of the chest, the pectoralis major and minor, and the axilla is completely cleared of all the lymph nodes. This operation is less frequently done at the present time.

Simple Mastectomy

This is the most common operation practised in Britain today. The breast is completely removed but the muscles are left giving a much more acceptable result with a normal anterior axillary fold. The incision (Fig. 11) is transverse so that the patient can wear a reasonably low neck or swim suit without embarrassment. Some surgeons combine this operation with a partial dissection of the axillary nodes and others leave the nodes. Postoperative radiotherapy to destroy any cancer which may remain in the lymph nodes or skin flaps is usually given.

Lumpectomy

As this descriptive word indicates the operation comprises a wide local excision of the lump in the breast. The operation is followed by radiotherapy in all cases as there is no information concerning involvement of the axillary nodes. This operation is not at present popular though further study may show its results to be no worse than full mastectomy. Unfortunately, even lumpectomy often results in quite a considerable deformity of the remaining breast.

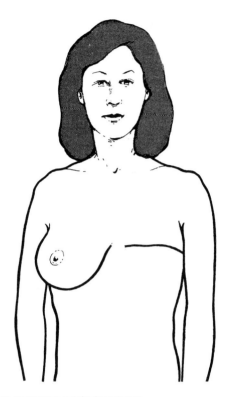

Fig 11   Modern transverse mastectomy scar

Mastectomy with Implant

There are technical difficulties with this operation in which a silicone filled implant is placed in the position of the breast which has been removed. It is not commonly performed in this country.

Postoperative Care of Breast Surgery

Many surgeons close a mastectomy wound with a continuous suture of nylon or other non-absorbable suture though some use interrupted sutures. The large skin flaps produce a lot of serous fluid after the operation and one or two suction (Redivac) drains are left in the wound and secured with a suture. The wound may be covered with Melolin or other non-adhesive dressing and Elastoplast but the transparent Op-Site dressing is becoming more popular. Mastectomy is a major operation and blood loss may be sufficient to require blood transfusion. The blood pressure and pulse rate need to be watched at regular intervals and a fall in blood pressure and rising pulse may indicate surgical shock requiring blood transfusion. The suction drains should be watched at frequent intervals to ensure that the vacuum is maintained. There is no set time for removal of the drains. They are removed when drainage stops and this may be up to seven or eight days in some cases. Too early removal of the drains will result in a collection of serous fluid which forms a lump called a seroma. If a seroma appears it is aspirated daily and if resistant to aspiration the drain may have to be replaced. The sutures are left for eight to ten days depending on the tension and the advice of the surgeon should be sought.

After dissection of the axillary nodes there is a tendency for shoulder movement to be uncomfortable or even painful. The arm is usually rested on a pillow for comfort but it is essential to encourage the patient to move the shoulder from the day following the operation and she should be able to comb and brush the back of her head by the third day.

There is no doubt that some women suffer a severe shock and depression following mastectomy. Eventual adjustment is nearly always complete but in some cases the patient is completely unable to accept the situation. Much depends on a sympathetic family and particularly husband. But the doctors and nurses must do their utmost to encourage the patient and to concentrate on the fact that she is now cured of the disease and able to return to her family, even though there must be some doubt in the surgeon's mind about permanent cure even in the most favourable cases. The widespread knowledge that breast cancer frequently recurs is a patent cause of serious anxiety and depression. It is essential that the patient should see her wound at an early stage. The longer this is put off the more difficult it becomes. An early visit from the appliance officer is essential. If the wound is tender at the time of discharge a temporary prosthesis made of wool must be fitted inside the brassière to give the patient confidence but the permanent prosthesis should be worn as soon as possible. The prosthesis is worn inside a normal bra. Modern prostheses are matched for shape and size. Some contain fluid which gives natural movement but patients need to be warned of the effect of pinning a broach accidentally to a fluid filled prosthesis. A swimming suit or bikini needs a pocket to contain the prosthesis as otherwise it may float out during swimming.

Adjuvant Therapy

The idea that a breast cancer has already been present for several years at the time of diagnosis has led to the idea that micrometastases are already present. It is therefore logical to give some generalised treatment immediately following mastectomy with the object of controlling these microscopic metastases while the operation removes the main bulk of the tumour. A number of trials of combined chemotherapy and hormone therapy are in progress at the present time. Early results are promising but it is too early to be dogmatic and these treatments are not yet routinely used following mastectomy.

Radiotherapy in the Primary Treatment of Breast Cancer

Radiotherapy is used in the treatment of the primary tumour when the surgeon considers it to be locally inoperable. This may be because of attachment to the chest wall or extensive involvement of skin.

Some patients refuse mastectomy and are given radiotherapy as the primary treatment.

In some parts of Europe, particularly France, radiotherapy is routinely used as the primary treatment. This is in the form of external radiotherapy supplemented by radiation from implanted radioactive material.

With the improvement of radiotherapeutic techniques and the obvious cosmetic advantages it seems likely that radiotherapy as the routine primary treatment will have an increasing role in the future.

Treatment of Advanced and Recurrent Breast Cancer

1   *Local Recurrence*

Local recurrence occurs in the axillary nodes and in the area of the skin flaps where it appears as nodules in the skin or subcutaneous tissue.

2   Distant Metastases

Metastases may occur almost anywhere but are common in the bones, liver, lungs, and brain. They may be found at the first consultation or appear after an apparently successful mastectomy.

There are three possible lines of treatment in disseminated disease:

Radiotherapy.   When a secondary deposit of cancer occurs in bone it usually causes pain. As the deposit of cancer spreads the bone may be so weakened that a fracture results. The common sites for this disaster are the weight bearing areas in the vertebrae and the neck and shaft of the femur. Fracture is accompanied by sudden severe pain and inability to stand. Deep X-ray therapy is used freely for bone secondaries. If the femur fractures the bone is splinted with an intramedullary nail (see Fig. 69) and radiotherapy given to control the cancer.

Radiotherapy is also used in some other sites including the brain.

Endocrine Therapy.   Some breast cancers are dependent on a particular hormone environment for their continued growth. Endocrine therapy makes use of this fact. In clinical practice the use of hormones is generally on a trial basis. In some units a premenopausal woman with metastases is treated by removal of the ovaries (oophorectomy) or by destroying ovarian function with radiotherapy.

However, in many units the patient is first treated with the agent called tamoxifen. If the tumour does not respond to the use of tamoxifen other hormones such as androgens (male hormone) may be used. Operations for removal of the adrenal glands and pituitary, which are the source of hormones, are now rarely used.

Chemotherapy.   In patients with advanced or recurrent disease, combination chemotherapy is used if radiotherapy and hormone therapy are no longer indicated.

Carcinoma of the Male Breast

The male breast is also subject to cancer and about 1 % of cases of breast cancer occur in the male.

Prognosis of Breast Cancer

The disease is unpredictable but the prognosis is generally better when the diagnosis is early. However, it is still a killer disease and

25 % of patients with stage 1 disease (lump in breast only) are dead within five years. When the axillary nodes are involved (stage 2) 50 % are dead in five years. In advanced cases only 10 % are alive in five years.

Hormone Induced Affections

Fibroadenosis

Fibroadenosis occurs in young women between the ages of 18 and 30. This disease goes by many other names including chronic mastitis and mastopathia. It presents as an exaggerated form of the cyclical changes which were described in the section on physiology. However, the premenstrual pain and lumpiness is sufficient to take the patient to her doctor and a single tender lump usually causes great anxiety. There may be a pale yellow or green discharge from the nipple. The management consists of strong reassurance. Hormone therapy is not normally advised.

Breast Cyst

In the premenopausal decade from 40 to 50 a patient may form a cyst in the breast. This presents a solitary lump and may be indistinguishable from a cancer. However, at the diagnostic aspiration the surgeon withdraws fluid and the lump disappears. All that is necessary is advice to attend again should another lump appear in the breast. Not all surgeons send the aspirated fluid for cytology unless it is blood stained. Recurrence may occur in another part of the breast up to the time of the menopause.

Breast Infections

Bacteria reach the breast through the ducts at the nipple. During lactation the bacteria encounter milk which is an ideal medium for growth. A lactating breast is most likely to develop a breast abscess but it is also seen in elderly women with retracted nipples.

Treatment of Breast Abscess

It is obvious that the baby cannot suckle from an infected breast so that supplemental feeding will be required. Stilboestrol is no longer used to inhibit lactation as it gives rise to an increased risk of deep vein thrombosis. The patient is given antibiotics and the abscess usually requires surgical drainage.

Mamillary Sinus

Sometimes a small abscess forms in a large duct near the nipple and discharges onto the skin near the edge of the areola causing a small discharging sinus called a mamillary sinus. This requires an operation in which the sinus and the diseased duct are excised.

Duct Papilloma

A duct papilloma is a small wart-like innocent tumour which occurs in one of the major ducts under the areola. The main symptom is a blood stained discharge from the nipple. Rarely these tumours become malignant. A duct papilloma is treated by removal of the duct in which it is growing.

Fibroadenoma

A fibroadenoma is a benign tumour of the breast which occurs from the menarche to the late twenties. The lump is hard and very mobile in the breast. The treatment is removal. It is a minor operation and the patient only needs to stay in hospital overnight.

9

Thyroid Gland

Anatomy (Fig. 12)

The thyroid gland is situated in the neck. It consists of two lobes which lie on each side of the trachea or windpipe and are connected by a narrow piece of gland called the isthmus which runs across the front of the trachea. Under the microscope it is seen to consist of millions of tiny spheres which are called acini or follicles. The follicles are lined by thyroid cells and contain a homogenous substance called colloid.

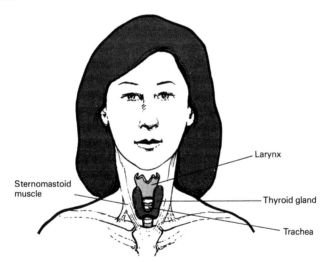

Fig 12 Position of the thyroid gland in the neck

Physiology

A small amount of iodine is necessary in the diet and this is provided by fish and dairy products. Iodine circulating in the blood is removed by cells of the thyroid gland. Very complicated chemical changes take place in the thyroid gland cells and the iodine is used to manufacture two substances called thyroxin and triiodothyronine, often referred to as T4 and T3. These chemical substances are hormones and are

57

stored in the follicles as colloid. When the body needs thyroid hormones they are released from the colloid into the blood stream.

Secretion of thyroxin is controlled by a hormone produced by the pituitary gland called thyroid stimulating hormone (TSH). When the blood level of thyroxin is too low the pituitary is triggered to secrete more TSH and this brings the blood level of thyroxin back to normal.

When a patient's thyroid function is normal she is said to be euthyroid. Increased function is hyperthyroidism which is also called thyrotoxicosis. Reduced function of the thyroid gland is called hypothyroidism. A special and severe form of hypothyroidism is myxoedema.

The hormones thyroxin and triiodothyronine regulate the metabolism of the body rather like a thermostat regulates the temperature of a central heating system. When the regulator is set too high the body functions are more active than normal (hyperthyroidism or thyrotoxicosis) and when it is too low the body functions are sluggish (hypothyroidism or myxoedema).

Investigations used in Thyroid Diseases

1   An X-ray of the neck is taken with the object of seeing if there is narrowing or displacement of the trachea by the enlarged thyroid.

2   The thyroxin (T4) circulating in the blood can be measured and the Free Thyroxin Index (FTI) calculated. The result of this test indicates if the patient is euthyroid or is suffering from hyper or hypothyroidism.

The physiologically active thyroxin circulates in the blood as free thyroxin. This accounts for less than 0.1 % of the circulating thyroxin. The rest is attached chemically to a globulin. This globulin is called thyroxin binding globulin (TBG). Certain drugs, particularly salicylates (aspirin) and Epanutin (a drug used in epilepsy) occupy the binding sites on the globulin and displace thyroxin. As a result the blood thyroxin will be low. The thyroxin binding globulin is raised in pregnancy and in patients taking the contraceptive pill. This may result in a high thyroxin level. Most request forms for blood thyroxin ask for information about drugs and the contraceptive pill to enable the biochemist to make an accurate interpretation of the result.

3   Radioactive scanning (Fig. 13) is used in some cases, particularly those in which there is a single lump in the thyroid gland. In this

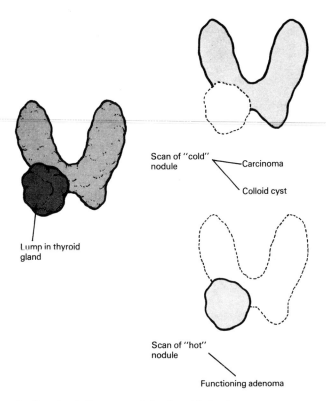

Scan of "cold" nodule — Carcinoma

Colloid cyst

Lump in thyroid gland

Scan of "hot" nodule — Functioning adenoma

Fig 13 Radioactive iodine scans of the thyroid gland

test the patient is given a minute amount of a radioactive isotope of iodine in a glass of water. The thyroid gland is unable to distinguish the radioactive isotope from ordinary iodine and it is taken into the gland in the usual way. When the radioactive iodine has been taken into the thyroid gland it is scanned by passing the probe of the scanner over the front of the neck and the distribution of iodine in the neck can be mapped out. If the lump does not take up iodine it is said to be 'cold'. This means that the lump is not active thyroid gland and it may be a cyst or a cancer of the thyroid. If the lump is found to be functioning it is said to be 'hot' and its activity usually suppresses activity in the rest of the thyroid.

The dose of radioactive iodine used is too small to have any adverse effect on the patient and also the isotope used has a very short half-life. The half-life of ^{131}iodine is eight days and this means that in this time half the radioactive isotope changes into ordinary iodine.

Diseases of the thyroid gland

Colloid Goitre

This is a disease which occurs at puberty when the body requirement for thyroid hormones is increased. If there is insufficient dietary iodine the thyroid cannot make enough thyroxin and the blood level falls. As a result there is an increase of pituatary TSH which causes some generalised enlargement of the thyroid gland. Colloid goitre does not require treatment. Removal of the enlarged thyroid gland (thyroidectomy) is contraindicated as it would further reduce the patient's ability to make thyroxin. Usually the condition improves without treatment and reassurance is all that is necessary. Iodine is sometimes given with benefit.

Adenoparenchymatous Goitre (Nodular Goitre)

In this condition the gland is replaced by nodules of varying size, usually with a great deal of colloid in the nodules and sometimes the production of a lump several centimetres in diameter and containing only colloid (a colloid cyst). The changes vary from a small nodule in one lobe to a great enlargement of both lobes. Sometimes the gland enlarges in a downward direction and extends behind the breast bone or sternum. This is called retrosternal goitre (Fig. 14).

The patient usually consults her doctor about a lump in the neck.

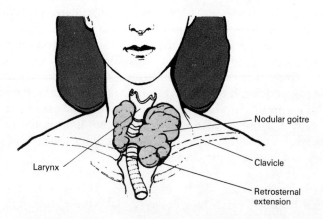

Fig 14   Displacement of the trachea by a large goitre partly retrosternal, on the left side

Diseases of the thyroid cause two types of symptoms, those due to an abnormal secretion of hormones and those caused by compression of structures adjacent to the thyroid lump or nodule. In uncomplicated nodular goitre thyroid function tends to be normal but in some cases, especially after thyroidectomy, the patient becomes hypothyroid. The mechanical effects of the enlarged gland are more important. The wind pipe (trachea) is often displaced and sometimes compressed. This may cause difficulty with breathing (dyspnoea) especially on exertion. Compression of the oesophagus is less often seen as it is placed behind the thyroid but some patients have minor difficulty with swallowing. When the thyroid enlargement extends behind the sternum (retrosternal goitre) it becomes wedged in a ring of bone comprising the sternum in front and the vertrabral column behind with the first rib on each side completing the circle. As the thyroid enlarges within this ring of bone the veins carrying blood from the head and neck to the heart are compressed and partly obstructed. This can be observed as the veins in the patient's neck become distended.

Treatment of Nodular Goitre

Nodular goitre is usually treated by thyroidectomy which is described later. As the patient is euthyroid there is no need for any special preparation.

The object of the operation is to remove the lump in the neck and to remove or prevent the onset of compression of important structures in the neck, particularly the trachea. Nodular goitre may also develop carcinoma or secondary thyrotoxicosis and thyroidectomy will prevent these complications.

Haemorrhage into a nodular goitre is rare but when it happens the sudden enlargement may cause sudden and dangerous compression of the trachea. This is another reason why surgeons advocate thyroidectomy in uncomplicated nodular goitre.

Hyperthyroidism (Thyrotoxicosis)

Thyrotoxicosis is a clinical condition caused by the production and circulation of an excess of the thyroid hormones, T_3 and T_4. It is now considered to be in the group of autoimmune diseases and due to the production and circulation in the blood of a substance which is called Long Acting Thyroid Stimulator (LATS).

There are two types of thyrotoxicosis:

1   *Primary thyrotoxicosis*

In this condition, which is also called Graves' disease, the gland is
uniformly enlarged. The excess of thyroid hormones causes an
increase in the metabolism of the cells of the body and a large variety
of clinical effects which are the easily recognisable disease known as
thyrotoxicosis or Graves' disease:

(a)   There is increased production of heat. The patient prefers the
cool of winter. The skin is warm and moist so that the body loses
more heat than normal. The increased cellular activity using up
energy causes the patient to have an excellent appetite but she loses
weight in spite of this. Most patients are women and young women
are affected more often than old, but the disease may occur at any age
and either sex.

(b)   Cardiovascular Effects.   The pulse rate is increased.
Nurses are usually asked to chart the pulse rate during sleep when
thyrotoxicosis is suspected because it remains elevated in sleep while
returning to normal in neurotic conditions which may mimic the
clinical symptoms of thyrotoxicosis. In severe cases the pulse may be
irregular because of abnormal contractions of the heart called atrial
fibrillation.

(c)   Nervous and Muscle Effects.   There are general signs of
nervousness. The patient is irritable and unable to sit still. She is also
emotionally unstable and may be quarrelsome with her husband and
family.

There is a fine tremor of the hands best demonstrated with the
hands outstretched.

The patient may complain of weakness and muscle fatigue and this
condition, which is called thyrotoxic myopathy, is seen to be caused
by wasting of certain muscles. The thigh and shoulder muscles are
most often affected.

(d)   Eye Signs.   Changes in the appearance of the eyes are a
characteristic feature (Fig. 15). The eyes are pushed forward in the
orbit by an excess of fluid which collects in the orbit behind the globe.
This is called exophthalmos. In addition to the obvious protrusion of
the eye it is possible to see the white sclera above the coloured iris of
the eye and in severe cases below as well. In severe cases the eye is
pushed so far forward that the patient is unable to close the lids to
cover the eye, which may be damaged during sleep causing ulceration
of the cornea. In other cases the eyes do not move normally and

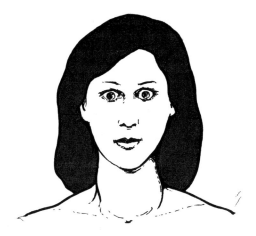

Fig 15 Exophthalmos seen in thyrotoxicosis

because the eyes are not properly lined up on looking to the side the two images are not superimposed in the brain and the patient sees double. This condition is called ophthalmoplegia. The severe cases of exophthalmos are called malignant exophthalmos and are a threat to normal sight.

(e) Miscellaneous. Menstrual abnormalities such as menorrhagia or amenorrhoea are sometimes seen. Diarrhoea is an occasional symptom.

2 Secondary Thyrotoxicosis

Some cases of nodular goitre develop the signs of thyrotoxicosis usually after the age of 40 years. This is called secondary thyrotoxicosis because it occurs in a gland which is already abnormal. Although the patient has similar symptoms and signs to those seen in primary thyrotoxicosis or Graves' disease the emphasis is different. The nervous symptoms and the eye signs are less marked but the cardiac signs are more prominent. Some patients present with a long standing nodular goitre and atrial fibrillation which gives the patient palpitations. An irregular pulse may be the only sign of hyperthyroidism.

Treatment of Thyrotoxicosis (Graves' Disease)

There are three different ways of treating primary thyrotoxicosis:

1   **Subtotal Thyroidectomy.**   In this operation the isthmus and most of the lateral lobes are removed. A small piece of gland at the back is left to produce thyroid hormones.

2   **Radioactive Iodine, ^{131}Iodine.**   The radioactive isotope ^{131}I is given to the patient. The advantage to the patient is that all he has to do is to take a drink of water containing the isotope. Obviously this is much more acceptable than a major operation. The object of the treatment is to give an amount of radioactive iodine which will be taken up by the thyroid and which will be sufficient to destroy enough of the gland to reduce its thyroxin production to normal. Prediction of the exact dose is difficult. An overdose will destroy the whole gland and make the patient severely hypothyroid and insufficient treatment will not relieve the thyrotoxicosis. The effect of radioactive iodine on the thyroid takes several months and it is usual to give the patient anti-thyroid drugs as described below during the period of time until the radioactive iodine becomes fully effective.

There has been some suggestion that radioactive iodine in this treatment dose, which is much higher than the dose used for diagnosis, might have some effect on the ovaries while circulating in the blood before being taken up by the thyroid gland. Radiation of the germ cells might result in the birth of congenitally abnormal babies. This particular form of treatment is therefore not used in women of child-bearing age.

3   **Antithyroid Drugs.**   The most commonly used drug is carbimazole which works by preventing the chemical formation of thyroxin in the thyroid gland. The disadvantages of antithyroid drugs in the treatment of thyrotoxicosis are:

(a)   It is necessary to continue the treatment for 18 months.

(b)   Rarely the drug suppresses the function of the bone marrow causing a fall in the white cell count which is called leucopenia. The patient becomes susceptible to infections of all kinds. The white blood cell count is measured at regular intervals so that the treatment can be stopped if the count falls.

(c)   The gland is inclined to enlarge and to become vascular especially if the dose of the drug is too high.

Treatment of secondary thyrotoxicosis

This condition is usually treated by thyroidectomy.

Lymphadenoid Goitre (Hashimoto's Disease)

This is an autoimmune disease in which the thyroid gland is gradually replaced with lymphocytes. As the normal thyroid tissue is replaced the gland enlarges slightly and the patient gradually becomes hypothyroid.

The patient is usually a middle-aged woman. If the surgeon suspects the diagnosis it can be confirmed by estimating thyroid antibodies in the blood. They are usually raised in lymphadenoid goitre. The surgeon may also do a needle or open biopsy.

Treatment

Surgical excision of the thyroid gland by thyroidectomy is contraindicated as it will only hasten the onset of myxoedema. The correct treatment is replacement therapy with thyroxin.

Carcinoma of the Thyroid Gland

Papillary and follicular carcinoma

Papillary and follicular carcinoma, so named because of their appearance under the microscope, may be grouped together as their behaviour is similar. Both occur in young people and sometimes in children. These are tumours of low malignancy and spread to lymph glands and by the blood stream to bone are late.

Treatment is by thyroidectomy, which may be total on one or both sides. The lymph glands in the neck are usually removed at the same operation.

Both of these tumours may be dependent for their growth on the pituitary hormone, thyroid stimulating hormone (TSH). The production of this hormone can be inhibited by giving the patient thyroxin for life following the operation. The prognosis is excellent.

Anaplastic carcinoma

Anaplastic carcinoma occurs in older patients and is much more malignant and usually fatal within a short time. A hard mass forms in the thyroid and the cancer quickly spreads outside the gland to invade surrounding structures:

1   Most important is invasion of the trachea which is narrowed causing shortness of breath and stridor. There is difficulty with inspiration accompanied by an audible crowing noise as the air passes through the narrow trachea.

2   The oesophagus is invaded causing severe difficulty with swallowing.

3   The recurrent nerves are invaded and paralysed. If the recurrent nerve is not functioning the vocal cord on that side does not move. This causes alteration of the voice and difficulty with breathing.

Treatment is usually by radiotherapy. Surgical excision is rarely possible because of spread to local structures such as the trachea. Sometimes the obstruction to the trachea has to be treated by making a tracheostomy below the obstruction.

Thyroidectomy

The operation of removal of the thyroid gland is called thyroidectomy. It may be total or partial. In the operation of partial thyroidectomy it is surgically convenient to leave the small piece of gland which is at the back. This ensures the preservation of the parathyroid glands which are placed behind the thyroid gland and within the capsule. In the operation of total thyroidectomy it is likely that all the four parathyroid glands will be removed so that the patient will develop tetany which will require treatment. The recurrent laryngeal nerves are also placed behind the gland on their way to the larynx.

Preoperative Treatment

In non-toxic cases there is no special preoperative preparation but toxic cases are treated with an antithyroid drug such as carbimazole until they are euthyroid. This is done on an outpatient basis and may take some months in a severe case. Carbimazole is inclined to make the thyroid gland very vascular and this presents difficulty at the operation. When the patient is euthyroid she is given Lugol's Iodine for ten days. This has the effect of making the gland less vascular so that the operation is easier.

When the pulse rate is very rapid it may be slowed by giving propranolol which acts directly on the nerve endings in the heart.

Some surgeons ask for an ENT opinion on movement of the vocal cords before the operation.

At the end of the operation a drain is left in the wound. This used to be a piece of corrugated rubber drain but many surgeons now use a suction drain such as a Redivae drain. The skin may be closed with clips but a subcuticular prolene suture is also used.

Postoperative Course and Complications

In a routine case the drain can be removed in 24 hours but it should not be removed if there is still drainage. The wound is closed with a layer of catgut sutures under the skin. This enables early removal of the clips or skin suture. Clips are generally removed at 24 and 48 hours and a continuous prolene suture can be taken out on the second or third day. Early removal of skin clips or sutures contributes to a good linear scar.

1 Haemorrhage. This dangerous complication of thyroidectomy takes place within the first few hours after the operation. The blood clots within the wound and the drains are not effective. As the mass of clot in the wound increases compression of the trachea results with respiratory distress and cyanosis. Death from asphyxia may result unless the compression is relieved urgently. If the patient's condition is serious it may be necessary to remove the wound sutures in the ward to take the pressure off the trachea. No anaesthetic is necessary. The skin clips or suture are removed. When the skin flaps are separated a vertical line of catgut sutures is seen approximating the muscles in the midline of the neck. Some of these must also be removed to release the blood clot compressing the trachea. There is no fear that there will be a gush of uncontrolled bleeding. When the emergency is over the patient is returned to the theatre for reclosure of the wound. It is a rare emergency and at the time of reclosure it is usually impossible to identify the bleeding point which was responsible.

It is wise always to have a suture and clip removal tray available at the bedside in the first 12 hours following thyroidectomy.

2 Injury to the Recurrent Laryngeal Nerve. The recurrent laryngeal nerves supply most of the muscles of the larynx which control the movement of the vocal cords. The vocal cords move during speech and also open during inspiration to allow the passage of

an increased flow of air. When a recurrent nerve is damaged the cord
on that side does not move and lies in a position near to the midline.
The voice is hoarse and the patient is unable to sing a high note. When
both nerves are damaged the cords lie close together in the midline
and the flow of air through the larynx is obstructed. The patient
makes a loud crowing sound on inspiration and may become
distressed, because of difficulty in breathing, and cyanosed. The
patient may die of asphyxia unless relieved by the operation of
tracheostomy in which a tube is placed in the trachea below the
larynx. As a temporary relief an endotracheal tube can be passed
through the larynx.

3 Damage to the Parathyroid Glands.   The parathyroid
glands are situated at the back of the thyroid gland and within its
capsule and are often damaged in total, but rarely in partial,
thyroidectomy. These glands secrete a hormone called parathormone
which controls the metabolism of calcium in the body. When the
level of parathormone is reduced the blood calcium falls. Calcium is
concerned with the sensitivity of nerve endings and when the calcium
level falls the nerve endings show increased sensitivity. Usually the
first symptoms concern the sensory nerves and the patient complains
of spontaneous abnormal sensations such as 'pins and needles' in the
hands and fingers. Later there may be spasms of muscles (tetany). If
the patient's face is tapped over the facial nerve the facial muscles
contract. This is called Chvostek's sign.

The immediate treatment of postoperative tetany is to restore the
level of the blood calcium with intravenous injection of 10 ml of 10 %
calcium chloride or calcium gluconate. This has an immediate effect
on the symptoms of tetany but has to be repeated as symptoms recur.

Maintenance treatment consists of giving 10–15 g of calcium
lactate daily by mouth to boost the blood calcium. Vitamin D2 is also
given in a dose of 100 000 units daily as this vitamin assists the
absorbtion of calcium from the intestine. The hormone parathormone cannot be given as replacement as it raises the blood
calcium by taking calcium from the bones which will eventually
become seriously decalcified.

10

The Salivary Glands

The salivary glands produce the saliva in the mouth. Saliva contains an enzyme called ptyalin which begins the digestion of starch but the main function of saliva is to lubricate the food and to make swallowing easier.

There are three main salivary glands but there are small glands throughout the lining of the mouth which produce saliva. The most important glands are the parotid and the submandibular salivary glands.

Parotid Gland (Fig. 16)

The parotid gland is situated on the side of the face in front of the ear and is familiar to most people as it is the gland which is involved by painful swelling in the virus infection called mumps. The gland drains through a duct which opens in the mouth opposite the 2nd molar tooth of the upper jaw on each side.

Bacterial infections from the mouth are occasionally seen, especially in children. This condition is usually due to an abnormality of

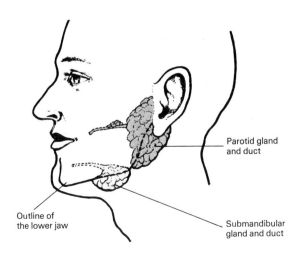

Parotid gland
and duct

Outline of
the lower jaw

Submandibular
gland and duct

Fig 16 Position of the parotid and submandibular salivary glands

the ducts which are wider than normal so that drainage is not free. Dilatation of the ducts is called sialectasis.

Stone formation in the parotid gland or duct is uncommon.

Tumours of the parotid are occasionally malignant — carcinoma of the parotid gland. The more common tumour is the salivary adenoma which was formerly incorrectly called a mixed parotid tumour.

Submandibular Gland

The submandibular salivary glands are situated partly under the middle third of the jaw on each side. The ducts drain into the mouth at orifices placed at each side of the fraenum of the tongue.

Stone formation and infection are the common affections in the submandibular salivary gland. The stones consist of calcium carbonate or phosphate and when large enough they block the lumen of a duct in the gland or the main duct outside the gland.

During mastication the salivary glands automatically secrete saliva. If there is a stone blocking the duct the saliva cannot escape and a painful swelling of the gland takes place every time the patient takes a meal.

Salivary tumours of the same type as seen in the parotid are seen rarely in the submandibular gland.

Radiography of the Salivary Glands

A plain film of the glands will usually show a stone if one is present. The duct system can be shown by cannulating the orifice of the submandibular or parotid duct and injecting radio-opaque contrast fluid, usually but erroneously called 'dye'. This is done in the X-ray department without anaesthetic.

Treatment

Operations on the salivary glands are not without risk of cosmetic problems and sometimes disaster.

The common operation on the parotid gland is for the removal of a salivary adenoma. The tumour is basically benign but will recur locally unless it is carefully removed with a margin of normal parotid gland. The operation is sometimes called superficial parotid lobectomy because the tumours usually arise in the superficial part of the gland. The surgical problem is that the facial nerve runs through the parotid gland to reach the muscles of the face and if any branch of the nerve is damaged during the dissection a part of the face will be paralysed permanently causing a serious cosmetic disability. If the nerve is stretched or damaged by retraction the same result will be seen but if the surgeon is confident that the nerve was not divided this paralysis will recover. Following excision a suction drain will be left in the wound for removal when serous drainage stops. If a major duct has been divided during the dissection there may be a considerable discharge of saliva from the drain but this may be expected to close spontaneously. If this complication is suspected it is better to leave the drain without suction so encouraging the drainage of saliva by the normal route.

The common operation on the submandibular gland is for stones. If a stone is lodged in the duct it can often be felt in the mouth and removed by an incision over it inside the mouth. Although this sounds an easy operation it is not always so and is usually done under a general anaesthetic. When the stone is in the gland, the gland has to be removed and this is done through an incision in the neck below the middle of the jaw. The main problem with this operation is that the branch of the facial nerve which supplies the muscle encircling the mouth loops down into the neck before rising to reach the mouth. If this nerve is cut during the operation a very damaging paralysis of the muscle around the mouth results. The mouth droops on the side of the lesion and the patient has difficulty in eating and saliva dribbles from the side of the mouth. There is no possibility of recovery but some help can be given by an operation in which the corner of the mouth is held up by a fascial sling which is inserted. Some surgeons are so concerned about this complication that they warn the patient about the possibility before doing the operation.

The wound drain is usually removed in 48 hours. As the whole gland is removed there is no possibility of a salivary fistula.

I I

Gallbladder and Bile Ducts

Anatomy and Physiology

The anatomy is shown in Fig. 17.

Bile is produced in the liver and excreted through the bile ducts. During fasting the muscular sphincter at the lower end of the bile duct is closed so that bile passes into the gallbladder where water is absorbed and the bile concentrated. When the patient takes a meal, the fat content causes the secretion of a hormone called cholecystokinin which makes the gallbladder contract. This raises the pressure within the duct system and the sphincter relaxes and bile flows into the duodenum to contribute to the process of digestion of food.

The important contents of bile are:

1 Bile Pigments

The red blood corpuscles of the blood function for about 100 days and then break down. The iron and protein is conserved by the body and used again for making more red blood corpuscles. The pigment is broken down and excreted by the liver as bile pigments. These give the bile its characteristic colour and also contribute to the colour of a normal stool.

2 Bile Salts

These are manufactured in the liver and are secreted in the bile. Bile salts are reabsorbed from the distal part of the small intestine and returned to the liver so that there is a circulation and conservation of bile salts. They have two important functions. One is concerned with the absorbtion of fat from the intestine. If bile salts are absent fat absorbtion is impaired and fat is passed in the stool. This is called steatorrhoea in which the stool is pale in colour, bulky and offensive. The second function is to keep a substance called cholesterol in solution. Cholesterol is present in normal bile and if the level of bile salts is reduced this substance comes out of solution to form a cholesterol gallstone.

72

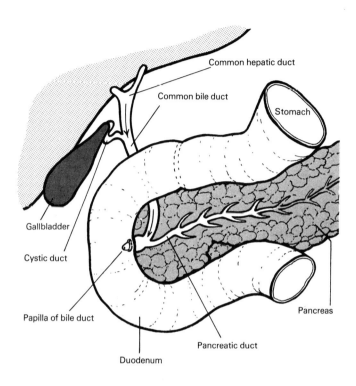

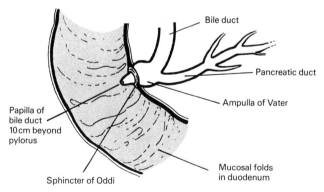

Enlargement to show detail of entry of bile and pancreatic ducts
into the duodenum

Fig 17 Anatomy of the gallbladder and bile ducts

Diseases of the Gallbladder and Bile Ducts

Gallstones

The most important disease is gallstones which form in the gallbladder. Initially they do not cause symptoms but complications are very likely after some time. Gallstones are becoming more common in this country and younger people are more often affected. The old saying that gallstone patients were 'fair, fat and 40' is not as true as it used to be. Gallstones in the gallbladder are often silent and discovered by accident. The symptoms of gallstones are the symptoms of complications. One complication is infection within the gallbladder. This is called cholecystitis and presents as an acute illness with severe upper abdominal pain particularly on the right side under the ribs and referred to the back or right shoulder blade. Vomiting and low fever are usual. If the cystic duct is obstructed the gallbladder may fill with pus. This is called an empyema of the gallbladder. Cholecystitis tends to settle with conservative treatment and antibiotics so that operation is not usually advised in the acute phase.

The second group of complications are caused by movement of the gallstones from the gallbladder.

1 Gallstone Colic. This is caused by strong contractions of the gallbladder attempting to push a stone from the gallbladder through the cystic duct to the common bile duct. The pain is felt in the central upper abdomen and is often accompanied by vomiting. The pain is very severe and patients often comment that it is worse than labour.

The pain usually lasts for about 4 to 6 hours and is so severe that the doctor is called. An injection of pethidine is usually given to relieve pain.

2 Migration of Stones into the Common Bile Duct. If stones lie freely in the bile duct they may not cause any symptoms. They are present in about 10 % of cases operated on for gallstones. However, the stones may become impacted and completely or partially obstruct the common duct. This is a serious complication as the bile cannot escape and the patient becomes jaundiced as a result of retention in the blood and tissue of bile pigments which continue to be manufactured. Liver and later renal failure may result so that relief is an urgent surgical requirement. Infection in the common duct is called cholangitis and adds to the seriousness of the condition.

A large stone sometimes migrates through the wall of the

gallbladder into the duodenum which lies alongside. In most cases this passes naturally in the stool but if it is large enough it can obstruct the intestine. This usually happens towards the lower end of the small intestine and is called 'gallstone ileus'. The patient is usually elderly and presents with acute intestinal obstruction.

Investigations of the Gallbladder

The gallbladder may be investigated by radiography but the tests depend on the excretion of the radio-opaque dye in the bile and X-rays cannot be done if the patient is jaundiced. It is useful to prepare the bowel as gas and faecal shadows may overlie the gallbladder and the department of radiology will advise about this. Plain films are usually taken but only about 10 % of gallstones are radio-opaque.

Oral Cholecystogram

The patient is given tablets of radio-opaque contrast medium in the evening. She attends for the X-rays about 14 hours later. This gives time for absorption of the contrast medium and its secretion by the liver into the bile. Finally it passes into the gallbladder and is concentrated sufficiently to show on a radiograph. This X-ray will show a functioning gallbladder and may show stones. There is no risk though some patients vomit.

Intravenous Choledochogram

In this test, which is designed to show the bile ducts as well as the gallbladder, the contrast medium is given by intravenous infusion over a period of half an hour. At the end of this time radiographs are taken which should show the common bile duct in addition to the gallbladder. There is a very slight risk attached to this investigation.

Obstructive Jaundice

Radiography has no place in obstructive jaundice. Often the surgeon will rely on clinical evidence but if there is doubt about the diagnosis other tests may be done.

Liver function tests are a group of blood tests that help to distinguish between obstructive and other forms of jaundice, particularly hepatitis.

Operations on the Gallbladder and Bile Ducts

Preoperative Preparation

If the patient is jaundiced there may be a defect in blood coagulation caused by the non-absorption of vitamin K which is fat soluble and not absorbed in steatorrhoea. To overcome this, the patient is given intramuscular injections of 10 mg of vitamin K twice daily for 48 hours before the operation. The second problem is renal failure occurring in jaundice. To overcome this an intravenous infusion is set up before the operation and about one litre of dextrose and saline is given in about one hour. During the operation the anaesthetist gives 20 ml of 10 % mannitol which acts as a diuretic. A catheter draining into a sterile bag is required as the diuresis occurs when the patient is anaesthetised and recovering.

Operation

The usual operation for gallstones is cholecystectomy or removal of the gallbladder. If there are stones in the common bile duct the duct is opened and the stones removed. The duct is then closed with sutures but a T-tube is left in place with the short arms of the T in the duct (Fig. 18). Using this technique, if the bile does not pass freely into the duodenum it will pass through the tube and be collected in a sterile bag. A second drain, often a small suction drain, is also left in the abdomen to drain away any bile which does escape.

If a stone is impacted in the sphincter at the lower end of the duct it may be necessary to open the duodenum to reach it and to incise the bile duct to get it out. This operation is called sphincterotomy or sphincteroplasty.

Postoperative Care

A gastric suction tube is not always necessary but if one is left in the stomach, an intravenous infusion will also be set up to provide fluid. The usual observations concerning postoperative shock and

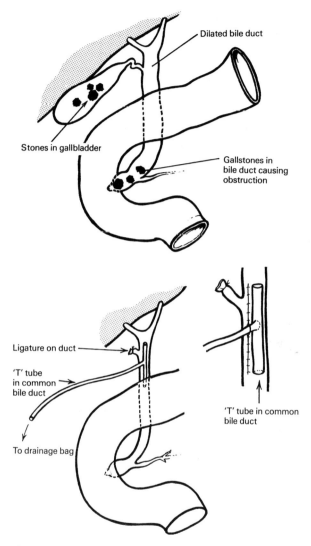

Fig 18 Cholecystectomy and exploration of bile duct for removal of stones

haemorrhage are made, i.e. quarter hourly observations of the blood pressure and pulse with less frequent observations as the patient's condition becomes more stable.

There are several tubes which require nursing care and observations.

The gastric drainage tube is attached to a drainage bag. The amount of gastric fluid is measured and charted.

The urinary output is measured and charted. In deeply jaundiced patients it is likely that a catheter will be in position and the bag is emptied and the contents measured and charted as ordered by the surgeon.

The T-tube drains into a similar bag and is emptied daily and the contents measured and charted.

It is obvious that when the T-tube is removed a small hole is left in the common bile duct. If the T-tube is removed in two or three days the bile will flow out of the hole in the bile duct and run all over the peritoneal cavity causing bile peritonitis. This is the reason that the T-tube is left in place for at least six days. By this time the body has made a track around the tube so that when it is removed any bile escaping from the bile duct runs along the track which is formed around the tube and reaches the skin surface. A dressing may be needed for a few days but the bile leak clears up in 24 to 48 hours provided the normal route for passage of bile into the duodenum is unobstructed. Surgeons vary in their exact timing but a postoperative choledochogram is asked for on about the 6th to the 10th day. In this test the patient is taken to the X-ray department and radio-opaque contrast medium is injected into the T-tube. This shows the bile duct and confirms that no stones have been left in the duct. It is important to exclude any air during this injection as an air bubble can be mistaken for a stone. If the duct is shown to be normal and with a free flow of the radio-opaque medium into the duodenum the T-tube is closed with a spigot or clamp the following day. Provided there is no leakage around the tube it can be removed on the following day.

12
Jaundice

Three types of jaundice are recognised. These are:

1 Haemolytic jaundice (sometimes called prehepatic jaundice);

2 Hepatocellular jaundice which is caused by disease of the liver cells (hepatic jaundice);

3 Obstructive jaundice, in which there is an obstruction to the flow of bile somewhere between the liver cells and the duodenum (post hepatic jaundice).

Normal Circulation of Bilirubin (Fig. 19)

Bile pigment is derived from the pigment which is normally present in the red blood corpuscles and to understand the different types of jaundice it is necessary to describe the natural process of destruction of the red blood corpuscles. The pigment in the red blood corpuscles is called haemoglobin and this is the substance to which oxygen gets attached for transportation to all parts of the body. These corpuscles are made in the bone marrow and live for about 100 days. They are destroyed in cells of the reticuloendothelial system, which are located in many parts of the body but mainly in the liver and spleen. When the haemoglobin is broken down the iron and protein parts are separated and recycled in the manufacture of new red blood corpuscles in the bone marrow. The pigment passes into the blood where it is attached to a protein – albumin – which is a large sized molecule which cannot pass into the urine. This explains the fact that bile pigment does not normally appear in the urine although it is circulating in the blood. This form of bilirubin is called haemobilirubin. When the pigment reaches the liver it passes through the liver cells or hepatocytes. Here it is separated from albumin and attached to glucuronic acid. This is called conjugated bilirubin or cholebilirubin and it passes out of the liver cells into the bile duct and so into the intestine where it is acted on by bacteria and converted to stercobilinogen. This is passed with the faeces but a small amount is absorbed into the blood stream and passed in the urine where it is called urobilinogen.

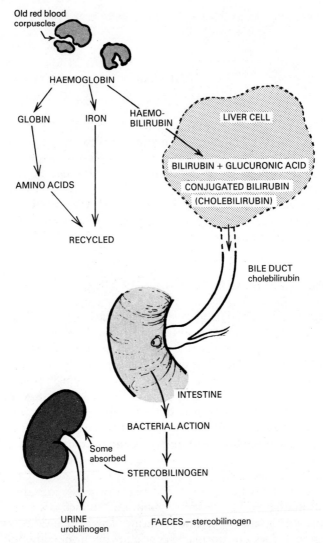

Fig 19 Normal bilirubin circulation

Haemolytic Jaundice (Fig. 20).

In haemolytic or prehepatic jaundice there is an excessive production of haemobilirubin. As this form of bilirubin has a large molecule it cannot pass through the kidney so that although the patient is jaundiced the urine does not contain bilirubin. This is called acholuric (no bile in the urine) jaundice.

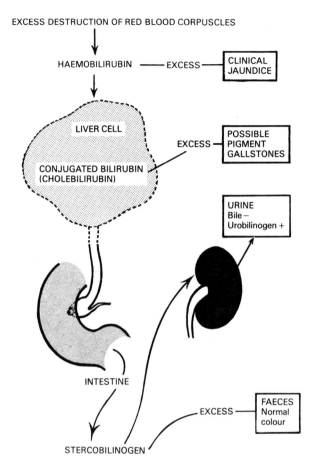

Fig 20 Bilirubin in haemolytic jaundice

There are a number of causes of haemolytic jaundice:

1   *Spherocytosis*

Normal blood corpuscles are biconcave but in the congenital condition known as spherocytosis or acholuric jaundice the blood corpuscles are spherical and break down much more quickly than normal ones. This leads to an increase in the amount of circulating haemobilirubin and clinical jaundice. A complication of the excessive amount of bile production is the formation of pigment gall stones. As most of the destruction of red corpuscles takes place in the spleen, the condition can be improved by removing the spleen (splenectomy) but this operation does not alter the basic abnormality of the red corpuscles which is present. If gallstones are present a cholecystectomy is also done.

2 Acquired Acholuric Jaundice

Sometimes, as a result of virus infections or the use of certain drugs, a patient may develop antibodies to his own red corpuscles and these antibodies cause an excessive breakdown of the red corpuscles similar to that seen in spherocytosis but the corpuscles are normal. This condition is rarely improved by splenectomy and is usually treated with steroids.

3 Incompatible Blood Transfusion

After large blood transfusions the transfused blood corpuscles may break up quickly and liberate enough haemobilirubin to cause a clinical postoperative jaundice.

Hepatocellular Jaundice (Fig. 21)

As the name implies this form of jaundice is caused by diseases which interfere with the function of the liver cells. The cells are unable to take up all the haemobilirubin which is in the blood so that the blood level of haemobilirubin is raised. Also, because of swelling in the liver, the minute bile canaliculi draining bile from the liver cells are partly obstructed so that the conjugated bilirubin cannot all pass into the bile ducts. The degree of obstruction varies but is often sufficient to cause the stools to be pale. The bile which cannot escape into the bile ducts is reabsorbed into the blood. As it is now in the form of conjugated bile it passes freely into the urine which is positive to tests for bile.

The main importance of hepatocellular jaundice to a surgeon is the distinction from obstructive jaundice which usually demands urgent surgical relief. The common causes are:

1 Virus Hepatitis

The two viruses which cause hepatitis are the hepatitis 'A' virus which causes acute infective hepatitis and hepatitis 'B' virus which causes serum hepatitis. Infective hepatitis has a characteristic clinical history with nausea and vomiting preceding the onset of jaundice. It is acquired by eating contaminated food. Serum hepatitis caused by hepatitis 'B' virus is spread by direct inoculation. It is possible to

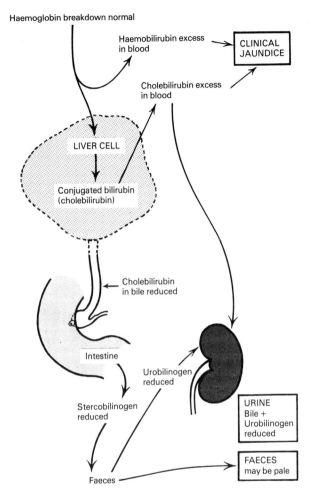

Fig 21 Bilirubin in hepatocellular jaundice

transmit the infection during transfusion but other injections can also be responsible, especially when the needle is not sterile as in drug addiction. It can also be transmitted during dental treatment if the dental surgeon is a carrier, and by tattooing. The disease is similar to infective hepatitis but the incubation is much longer, about 100 days, and the infection more dangerous. The antigen can be identified in the blood and is called Australia antigen. Technicians and nurses can get infected from accidental injuries and special precautions are taken with blood samples from infected patients. Surgeons need to take special precautions if the Australia antigen is present in the patient's blood.

If anyone of the staff gets an accidental prick or other injury or receives a splash of fluid in the eye there is a serious risk of infection. The Public Health Laboratory carries an effective hyperimmune globulin which should be given in such cases.

2   Cirrhosis

Some cases of cirrhosis of the liver may reach an advanced stage with jaundice before coming to hospital and these may clinically resemble obstructive jaundice.

Obstructive Jaundice (Fig. 22)

The patients with obstructive jaundice comprise most of the surgical cases. The bile ducts may be obstructed within the liver where the

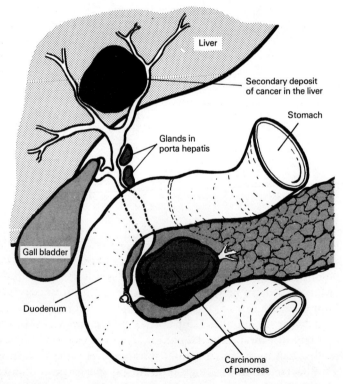

Fig 22   Three causes of jaundice through compression in the bile duct A stone blocking the duct is another common cause

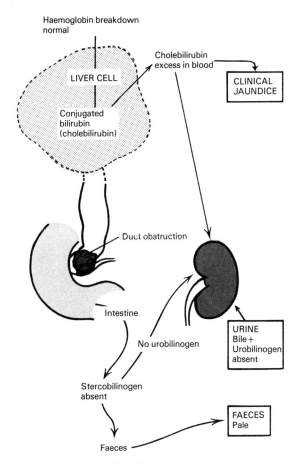

Fig 23 Bilirubin in obstructive jaundice

most common cause is compression by a metastasis. In the bile duct, compression may be outside the bile duct, in the wall of the duct, or within the lumen of the duct. Two common causes are a stone inside the duct and a carcinoma of the pancreas compressing the duct from the outside.

In obstructive jaundice the bile passes through the liver cells and is converted to its conjugated form (Fig. 23). This is reabsorbed into the blood stream causing clinical jaundice because the normal route into the bile duct is blocked. The urine contains bile because of the excess of cholebilirubin in the blood. As the bile is not entering the duodenum the faeces are pale in colour.

Nursing Observations in a Jaundiced Patient

Patients with jaundice are often depressed and need more than usual encouragement.

The usual observations of pulse, blood pressure and temperature are made.

The progress or natural relief of obstruction may be to some extent judged by the colour of faeces and urine and these should always be noted and reported. The return of colour to the faeces would indicate that an obstruction had ceased to be complete. There is a risk of renal failure and collection, measurement and charting of urinary output are important observations in a patient who is jaundiced.

Investigation of a Case of Jaundice

The clinical history and physical signs may leave the surgeon in no doubt as to the pathological diagnosis in a case of jaundice. However, many cases are difficult and need investigation. The surgeon needs to know if the case is one of obstructive jaundice. If it is he needs to know the exact cause before undertaking an operation for its relief.

1   Liver Function Tests

A group of blood tests can be done to assess liver function. Between 5 and 10 ml of blood is taken and transferred to a sterile bottle and allowed to clot. Albumin is solely made in the liver and in cases with an impaired liver function the blood albumin is low. An abnormal liver also produces abnormal globulins and these may be above the normal level giving a normal total protein but with too much globulin and not enough albumin.

Certain enzymes produced by the liver cells are present in abnormal amount in hepatitis but are normal in obstructive jaundice. One commonly used test is the aspartate amino transferase which is raised in hepatitis.

Alkaline phosphatase is an enzyme which is normally present in bile. In obstructive jaundice the blood level is raised because the passage of alkaline phosphatase from the blood to the duodenum is blocked. The blood level remains normal in hepatitis.

2   Ultrasonic Scanning

In this technique ultrasound waves are passed into the liver. The ultrasound echoes from solid areas such as metastatic deposits. Fluid-containing parts of the liver are transonic and so large ducts resulting from obstruction can be identified on the scan.

3   Isotope Scanning

In this study the patient is given an intravenous injection of a radioisotope of a substance called technetium which has been chemically attached to a colloidal form of sulphur. A colloidal solution consists of very tiny particles. All particles are removed from the blood by cells of the reticuloendothelial system and as most of these are in the liver 85 % of the isotope is taken up by the liver. Technetium remains radioactive for a very short time. (The half life is six hours which means that every six hours the activity is reduced by half.) The liver is scanned 15 minutes after the injection and defects more than 2 cm in diameter are usually identified.

4   Percutaneous Transhepatic Choledochography (Fig. 24)

If it is already suggested that there is obstruction to the bile ducts and resulting dilatation of the intrahepatic ducts this investigation can

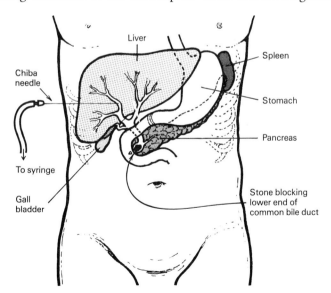

The Chiba needle has been placed in the lumen of a dilated intrahepatic duct
Following the injection of contrast medium the ducts will be seen and the
stone blocking the lower end of the bile duct will be outlined

Fig 24   Percutaneous transhepatic choledochogram

help to decide the cause of the obstruction. Under local anaesthetic it is possible to place a needle into a bile duct and to display it by injecting radio-opaque contrast medium.

The patient goes to the X-ray department. Local anaesthetic is given and a very fine, springy needle is passed into the liver. Radio-opaque contrast medium is injected and the liver viewed on a television screen. If injected contrast enters a blood vessel it is seen to flow away quickly with the blood and injection into the liver substance remains as a patch of dye. When dye enters a bile duct it is obvious on the screen. Bile is too viscous to aspirate through the needle for confirmation. Once the needle is safely in a duct an injection of contrast medium is made and the cause of the obstruction is usually seen.

The danger of this investigation is tearing the liver accompanied by bleeding or leak of bile from a dilated duct along the needle track into the peritoneal cavity causing bile peritonitis. To avoid this the patient is asked to stop breathing while the needle is being moved by the radiologist and to breathe with shallow respirations once it is in position. The investigation has been made much safer by the introduction of the very fine Chiba needle.

Because of these rare complications patients are carefully watched for signs of bleeding or bile peritonitis after return to the ward. Observations are made on the pulse and blood pressure at half hour intervals. Bile peritonitis usually causes severe abdominal pain and if the patient complains of this the doctor should be informed.

ERCP. This stands for Endoscopic Retrograde Cannulation of the Common bile duct and Pancreatic duct. A special side viewing gastroduodenoscope is passed into the duodenum. The bile duct papilla is found and a special catheter can usually be manipulated through the papilla into the bile duct or the pancreatic duct. If a tumour of the papilla (usually called an ampullary carcinoma because of its origin from the Ampulla of Vater) is found, a biopsy can be taken. If a catheter is passed through the papilla it is possible to inject radio-opaque contrast medium and to show any abnormality of the duct such as a stricture or bile duct stones. The Chiba needle investigation is easier and is more commonly used as the first investigation.

This technique can also be used to enlarge the opening of the bile duct into the duodenum so allowing the passage of bile duct stones obstructing the common bile duct. In this operation a diathermy wire is passed into the bile duct and used to cut and enlarge the opening. This operation may be complicated by bleeding and after return to the ward it is necessary for the nurse to make careful observations of the vital signs and to report any rise in pulse and fall in blood pressure which might indicate internal bleeding.

13

Pancreas

Anatomy

The pancreas lies across the upper abdomen with the right-hand end placed within the C of the duodenum. The gland stretches across the back of the abdomen in front of the aorta and vena cava to reach the spleen on the left hand side. It lies behind the stomach. The pancreatic duct joins the bile duct at the Ampulla of Vater and pancreatic juice is discharged through the bile duct papilla into the duodenum (Fig. 17).

Physiology

The pancreas is a gland which has an exocrine secretion which discharges through the duct into the duodenum, and endocrine secretions which discharge direct into the blood.

Exocrine Secretion of the Pancreas

The pancreas secretes about 1 litre of fluid or juice each day. The juice passes through the pancreatic duct and mixes with the food in the duodenum. Its function is to break down the various substances of food into simple products which can be absorbed by the intestine. The juice contains bicarbonate which gives an environment in which pancreatic enzymes can work and digest food to best advantage. Enzymes are important in many physiological processes. Some work best in acid and others in alkaline medium. They assist and accelerate chemical reactions.

Protein Digestion

The basic unit of protein is an amino acid. If this can be thought of as a link in a chain then several links of the chain joined together is called a polypeptide and a protein is made from polypeptides. The particular type of protein is determined by the particular amino acids from which it is constructed.

The pancreas secretes enzymes called trypsinogen and chymotrypsinogen. They are inactive in this form but as soon as they reach the duodenum they are activated by contact with an enzyme called enterokinase which is secreted in the duodenum. In this remarkable way the enzyme does not digest the pancreas but becomes active when it reaches the safe area of the duodenum. The activated hormones are called trypsin and chymotrypsin and they convert the long chain polypeptides into shorter chains and finally into single units or amino acids.

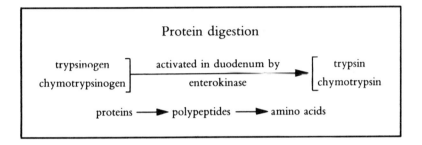

Fat Digestion

Fat is ingested in the form of neutral fats in which glycerol is attached to three fatty acids and is called a triglyceride. The pancreas secretes an enzyme called lipase which releases some of the fatty acids. The result is some free fatty acids and the remaining glycerol attached to two or one fatty acid. These compounds are called mono- and di-glycerides. The bile salts in the bile have the effect of emulsifying fat globules in the food and this conversion of fat droplets into very tiny globules makes it easier for the lipase to reach the fat and act on it. Without bile in the intestine, as in obstructive jaundice, fat digestion is greatly reduced.

After digestion the monoglycerides join with fatty acids and bile salts to form an aggregate which is called a micelle. This compound is much smaller than the emulsified fat globule and is in a form which is capable of absorption through the intestinal mucosa.

Digestion of Carbohydrates

Starch and glycogen are two important types of carbohydrate in food. Starch occurs in plants which are used as food and glycogen is a

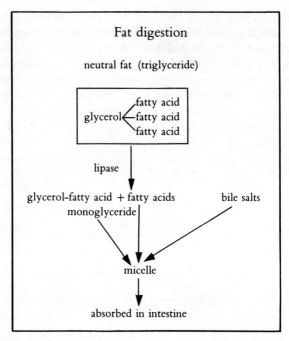

carbohydrate which is present in animal tissues. It is present in human tissue and is stored in the liver.

The basic unit of a carbohydrate is a substance called a monosaccharide and glucose and galactose are important examples. These basic units are connected in chains to form polysaccharides.

Starch is composed of straight chains in which the individual links are glucose and glycogen is a branched chain of glucose molecules.

The pancreas secretes an enzyme called amylase which breaks down polysaccharides such as starch into glucose which is absorbed by normal intestine.

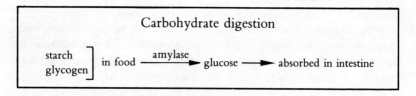

Control of Secretion of the Pancreas

When food enters the duodenum two hormones are produced in the mucosa of the duodenum. These are called secretin and pancreozymin. They pass from the mucosa into the blood stream and when they reach the pancreas it is stimulated to secrete its enzyme-containing juice. In this way the pancreas only produces digestive enzymes when food is passing through the duodenum and ready for digestion.

Morphine and codeine cause spasm in the muscle surrounding the duct as it passes through the duodenum and prevent the escape of pancreatic juice. On the other hand the muscle relaxes if the patient is given atropine or propantheline bromide (Pro-Banthine) and these drugs assist the flow of bile and pancreatic juice into the duodenum.

Endocrine Secretion of the Pancreas

The pancreas is also an important endocrine gland. When the gland is examined with a microscope small groups of cells which secrete hormones are seen between the glands. These groups of cells were first seen and described by Langerhans and are called Islets of Langerhans. Three hormones are produced by different cells in the Islets:

1 α-cells secrete a substance called glucagon. Glucagon acts on the glycogen which is stored in the liver and breaks it down into glucose which passes into the blood stream causing a rise in the blood sugar, i.e. the opposite effect of insulin.

2 β-cells are the source of insulin. The β-cells account for 75 % of the islet cells. Insulin promotes the absorption of glucose into the tissues from the blood and so causes a drop in the blood sugar.

3 δ-Cells are thought to secrete gastrin which is also secreted by the stomach.

Acute Pancreatitis

Acute pancreatitis is a condition in which the enzymes trypsinogen and chymotrypsinogen are activated into trypsin and chymotrypsin in the pancreas instead of in the duodenum. Digestion of the blood vessel walls causes retroperitoneal haemorrhage which may be severe enough to cause shock. All the enzymes secreted by the pancreas escape behind the peritoneum and also into the peritoneal cavity. The effect of the proteolytic enzymes in the peritoneal cavity is to cause paralytic ileus. Pancreatic lipase releases fatty acids from the neutral fat in the omentum. The fatty acids combine with calcium to form soaps which give a characteristic appearance in the peritoneal cavity where patches of white soaps are seen on the normal yellow fat. This appearance, which is characteristic of pancreatitis, is known to surgeons as fat necrosis. The exact cause of the activation of pancreatic enzymes in the pancreas is unknown.

Pancreatitis is commonly associated with gallstones and cholecystitis, and recurrence of acute pancreatitis can be prevented by removal of the inflamed gallbladder. Another and smaller group of cases of pancreatitis are associated with alcoholism. There remain a group of about 20 % of cases in which no clear association is seen and these are called idiopathic.

There is a very wide spread of severity of acute pancreatitis. Some cases are quite mild and resolve in a few days but at the other extreme the patient may die of haemorrhagic shock and the effect of ileus. In some of the more severe cases a collection of pancreatic fluid localises in front of the pancreas and this is called a pseudocyst of the pancreas. A true cyst has a capsule but in this condition the pancreatic fluid is localised by the reaction of the surrounding tissue and having no true capsule is called a pseudocyst. In other more severe cases the body of the pancreas dies and forms a slough because its blood vessels have been destroyed. This dead tissue easily becomes infected to cause a pancreatic abscess. The treatment of these two serious complications of pancreatitis is illustrated in Fig. 25.

Treatment of Acute Pancreatitis

There is no surgical treatment of acute pancreatitis but some patients are operated on because the surgeon is in doubt about the diagnosis and fears missing some other emergency such as a perforated ulcer which requires urgent surgical closure.

In acute pancreatitis the serum amylase is considerably raised. To do this test 5 ml of blood is taken in a heparinised bottle. Levels above 1000 units are diagnostic of pancreatitis.

Nursing a patient with acute pancreatitis can be a challenging experience as the patient may remain very ill for some days. The basis of treatment is to try to minimise the secretion of pancreatic enzymes and to encourage their flow to the duodenum. An indwelling gastric tube is used to keep the stomach empty. As the patient has ileus the stomach tends not to empty and fills with gastric and duodenal secretions. In addition it is necessary to minimise the passage of gastric contents to the duodenum as this results in the stimulation of the pancreas through the action of the duodenal hormones pancreozymin and secretin. The second mainstay of treatment is the use of drugs such as atropine and propantheline bromide (Pro-Banthine) which

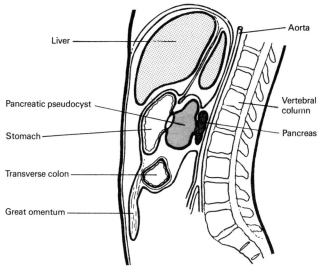

Operation for pancreatic pseudocyst
The stomach is opened and its back wall opened into the pseudo cyst
The two structures are sutured together to make a permanent opening from
the pseudocyst into the stomach. The front of the stomach is then closed

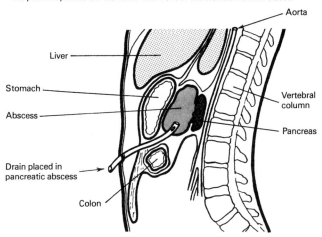

A pancreatic abscess is drained with a tube drain. The is removed when
drainage stops. Usually two to three weeks

Fig 25   Complications of acute pancreatitis

relax the muscle at the opening of the pancreatic and bile ducts and so
assist the flow of juice containing enzymes from the pancreas.
The treatment therefore consists of:

   I   Intravenous infusion to replace fluid and electrolytes lost and also to give blood as necessary in the treatment of haemorrhagic shock.

2   A gastric tube to allow the aspiration of gastric fluid so preventing its entry into the duodenum.

3   Atropine or propantheline bromide to encourage the flow of juice from the pancreas.

4   Relief of pain. Morphine and its derivatives are not used as they cause spasm of the muscle surrounding the duct as it passes into the duodenum and although useful for pain relief has an effect opposite to that of atropine and prevents the flow of pancreatic juice into the duodenum. Pethidine is the drug usually given for pain in pancreatitis.

5   Two drugs have had some popularity in recent years. Trasylol is an inhibitor of trypsin and should stop its proteolytic action. Glucagon is a drug which mobilises glycogen and converts it into glucose so raising the blood sugar. It also suppresses gastric function and should therefore inhibit the secretin mechanism and reduce pancreatic enzyme secretion. Both of these drugs have had extensive trial but at the present time there are no hard data to support their use.

Tumours of the pancreas

There are a few benign tumours of the pancreas called cystadenomas but the usual pancreatic tumour is a malignant adenocarcinoma arising from the secretory cells of the pancreas.

Carcinoma of the pancreas

Carcinoma of the head of the pancreas presents in the same way as a carcinoma of the Ampulla of Vater but is much more deadly and can rarely be cured by resection. Both cause obstruction of the common bile duct. The patient goes to the doctor with signs of obstructive jaundice but without pain. Pain accompanying jaundice is usually due to gallstones but painless jaundice is a very serious symptom often indicating a carcinoma obstructing the common bile duct.

Carcinoma of the Ampulla of Vater is less malignant and spreads more slowly to reach the vital structures outside the pancreas. Carcinoma of the head of the pancreas becomes inoperable at an early stage. It infiltrates the superior mesenteric artery which supplies all the

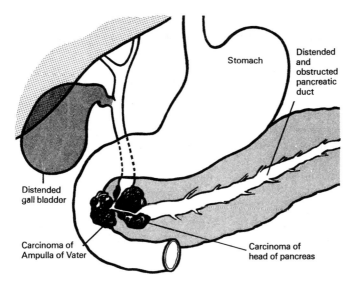

Malignant obstruction of the common bile duct causing obstructive jaundice

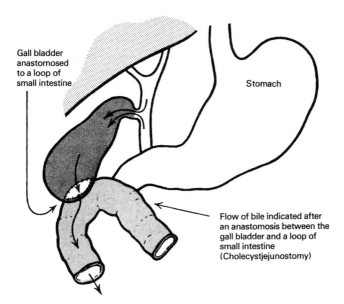

Fig 26 Palliative treatment of malignant obstructive jaundice

small intestine and also the important structures such as the aorta and vena cava which lie at the back of the pancreas. Even if it is possible to resect a carcinoma of the head of the pancreas recurrence is almost inevitable and most surgeons reserve resection and an attempt at cure for patients with a carcinoma of the Ampulla of Vater.

Most patients with these cancers complain of weight loss. This is because obstruction of the bile and pancreatic ducts reduces fat digestion and absorption (steatorrhoea).

Carcinoma of the body of the pancreas is even more difficult to diagnose and usually presents with severe back pain due to spread of the tumour to the structures at the back of the pancreas. Resection is very rarely possible. All cases of pancreatic cancer spread to lymph nodes and to the liver causing liver metastases.

Treatment of Carcinoma of the Head of the Pancreas

Most cases are explored after the routine preparation required for a patient with obstructive jaundice. Resection is rarely done but the patient is palliated by making an anastomosis between the very dilated gallbladder and a loop of small intestine so relieving the jaundice. Patients treated in this way live in reasonable comfort for up to a year (Fig. 26).

Treatment of Carcinoma of the Ampulla of Vater

At exploration these cases are also often found to be inoperable and are palliated by a short circuit operation as in the case of a carcinoma of the pancreas. However, the surgeon may occasionally elect to resect the head of the pancreas. This is a difficult and complicated operation and requires a difficult reconstruction after the resection (Whipple, Fig. 27). Following a Whipple operation the patient will return to the ward with at least three drains from the abdomen. One is a T-tube which traverses the biliary-intestinal anastomosis and the other drains the pancreatic duct through the intestine. These drain into sterile drainage bags. There will also be at least one suction drain in the peritoneal cavity. The immediate postoperative observations are the vital signs, pulse and blood pressure.

The patient will be given intravenous fluids and in some cases, when there is delay in return of intestinal function, intravenous feeding can be given. About the fifth day the suction drains can be removed but they should be left if drainage is still present. On the

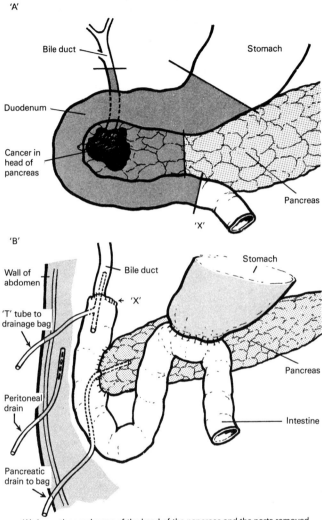

'A' shows the carcinoma of the head of the pancreas and the parts removed in the Whipple operation

'B' shows reconstruction. The cut end of intestine 'X' is anastomosed to the bile duct and the anastomosis splinted with a 'T' tube

A second drain splints the anastomosis between the pancreas and intestine

Fig 27 Whipple's operation for cancer of the pancreas

tenth day the patient is taken to the X-ray department and radio-opaque contrast injected into the T-tube and pancreatic drain. If these X-rays show that there is no anastomotic leak the drains can be removed.

Postoperative patients with pancreatic cancer are usually ill because of deep jaundice and malnutrition. A particularly sympathetic approach to the postoperative care is needed. The vital signs are observed at frequent intervals. Internal bleeding should not be a problem if the patient has been properly prepared with vitamin K. The particular postoperative problem in deeply jaundiced patients is renal failure. The patient will have been given a diuretic during the operation and will return from the theatre with a catheter in the bladder. Accurate measurement and charting of the urinary output is important and if the urine output is reduced the surgeon may decide to give a further diuretic. The patient will also have a gastric tube on drainage and an intravenous drip which needs the usual routine attention and charting.

There will probably be a drain in the abdomen to drain any leakage of bile from the anastomosis and, at the discretion of the surgeon, this will be removed after four or five days though it will be left longer if drainage of bile continues.

Islet Cell Tumours

The cells of the Islets of Langerhans normally secrete hormones and tumours arising in these cells secrete hormones in excessive quantity. The most common tumour secretes insulin and causes symptoms which result from a low blood sugar (hypoglycaemia).

14

The Oesophagus

Anatomy and Physiology

The oesophagus begins at the level of the lowest part of the larynx (voice box) which can easily be felt in the middle of the neck. It is a continuation of the pharynx and is a tube about 40 cm (10 inches) long which carries the food down through the chest and through the diaphragm to reach the stomach. Food which is eaten has at this time only been processed by munching and by the addition of saliva which has the function of lubrication. The food is often hard and may contain bone fragments which are accidentally swallowed. The lining of the oesophagus therefore needs to be strong and is virtually the same as skin. Bone spicules and sharp foreign bodies may penetrate the oesophagus but the strong lining makes this serious accident very unusual. When food enters the oesophagus it is transferred through the long tube to the stomach by a coordinated contraction of the muscle of the oesophagus behind the bolus of food at the same time as relaxation of the muscle in front. This process, which is called peristalsis, is used to transmit food throughout the whole gastrointestinal tract from the pharynx to the anus. Although it is useful to know that the oesophagus is 25 cm in length it is of more practical value to know that it begins about 15 cm (6 inches) from the incisor teeth and ends in the stomach about 40 cm (16 inches) from the incisor teeth. This information is useful in passing gastric tubes and endoscopes and enables the operator to know the location of the tip of the tube or endoscope by observing the length of tube which has been passed.

The oesophagus runs through the chest and is surrounded by vital structures. At the upper end the trachea is in front and after this has divided into two tubes called bronchi which pass laterally into each lung, the heart lies in front. The aorta comes out of the left ventricle at the top of the heart and arches back to run down through the chest as the thoracic aorta. As it arches it is so close to the oesophagus that it indents the left side of the oesophagus and this can be seen on barium X-ray of the oesophagus. At the lower end the oesophagus lies between the heart and aorta. These anatomical facts account for the difficulty of resecting tumours of the oesophagus which become attached to vital structures at an early stage and become inoperable.

Surgeons often refer to the three thirds of the oesophagus. The main bronchus and the main blood vessels to the lung form a pedicle to the lung about 7 cm (3 inches) in length. The part of the oesophagus opposite the lung root is called the middle third with the upper third above and the lower third below.

At rest the oesophagus is relaxed and contains a little air. This is an important fact as penetrating injury to the oesophagus or a leaking anastomosis is characterised by leakage of air which can easily be seen on an X-ray.

Proximal Oesophageal Sphincter

Anyone who has passed a tube or endoscope will know that it is difficult to get the tube from the pharynx into the oesophagus. Once this obstruction is overcome the tube passes easily to the stomach. There is no obvious difference in appearance at the site of the proximal sphincter but the muscle of the oesophagus at the upper end is normally contracted so that the lumen is closed. This prevents air which the patient is breathing from passing into the oesophagus where it would soon reach the stomach and cause discomfort and distension. It also has some effect in arresting the passage of fluid which has refluxed from the stomach and which might be spilled over into the trachea if it got above the oesophagus.

Gastro-Oesophageal Reflux

Food and drink which reaches the stomach does not normally reflux back into the oesophagus except in the act of vomiting. There are three mechanisms which prevent reflux:

1   There is a weak sphincter in the wall of the lower 3—4 cm of the oesophagus which is very similar to the sphincter at the upper end. It cannot be seen as a part of the oesophagus which has a different appearance but it remains contracted except during swallowing.

2   The acute angle at which the oesophagus enters the stomach is thought to be the most important mechanical factor preventing reflux and re-establishing this angle is the important part of most successful operations for reflux (Fig. 33).

3   The last 5 cm of the oesophagus is below the diaphragm. This last part of the oesophagus is subjected to positive intra-abdominal pressure and this probably keeps the lumen closed.

Symptoms of Oesophageal Diseases

Most of the diseases which affect the oesophagus cause difficulty in swallowing. If the oesophagus becomes narrow as a result of a malignant growth the patient complains that food will not pass down to the stomach but sticks at a point which he indicates with some confidence but which does not often coincide with the actual site of the obstruction. Non-malignant obstructions usually have a longer history and progress more slowly than the malignant cases.

Oesophageal pain is felt in the centre of the chest or back. It is usually caused by inflammatory changes which result from the reflux of gastric contents into the oesophagus. Many patients in middle age who have oesophageal pain are diagnosed as suffering from cardiac pain and nowadays are sometimes subjected to coronary arteriogram. Such patients with normal coronary arteriograms usually have oesophagitis.

Special Investigations

Patients with oesophageal symptoms are studied by barium swallow examination. The radiologist can watch the progress of barium down the oesophagus and also see if it refluxes back from the stomach. Abnormalities of the surface such as a cancer can readily be diagnosed.

Endoscopy is also used to examine the oesophagus. It has the advantage over radiology that a fragment of abnormal tissue can be removed for histology and specimens can also be collected from any lesion for cytological studies.

Carcinoma of the Oesophagus

About half the cases of oesophageal cancer occur in the lower third. Histologically these tumours are epitheliomata which are the same tumours as occur in skin. At the lower end some tumours are derived from stomach cells and are adenocarcinomata. The distinction is important as adenocarcinoma is resistant to radiation but epithelioma is sensitive and radiotherapy may be considered as a possible form of treatment.

Spread of Oesophageal Cancer

Local spread is to adjacent organs. In the case of the oesophagus the adjacent organs are of vital importance to life and early spread often makes resection impossible. The tumour may be attached to the aorta, to the pericardium which is the sac enclosing the heart, to the lung or its vessels and bronchi.

Tumours of the lower third are inclined to spread by lymphatic vessels to lymph nodes in the abdomen but tumours in the upper part of the oesophagus spread by lymph vessels towards the neck.

Blood stream spread is late but metastases may occur in liver, bone or lungs.

Diagnosis of Oesophageal Cancer

The outstanding symptom is progressive dysphagia, (difficulty in swallowing). The patient complains that food sticks in the gullet and is usually regurgitated. The symptom is progressive so that increasingly small pieces of food stick and finally water and saliva cannot pass down the oesophagus. At this stage water and saliva are regurgitated into the pharynx causing the patient to cough as the fluid falls into the larynx. Patients with this complication inhale infected fluid and mucus and this causes inhalation pneumonitis (inflammation of the lungs) and death. The lack of nutrition is soon evident and most patients have lost a lot of weight by the time they reach a hospital consultation. Some are emaciated.

In a suspected case the diagnosis is confirmed by X-ray and endoscopy when samples can be taken for histology and cytology.

Treatment of Oesophageal Cancer

The treatment may be curative or palliative. Attempts at cure are usually by surgical resection but some cases can be cured by radiotherapy and this is indicated if the tumour is an epithelioma and therefore sensitive to radiation and at the same time the patient is judged not strong enough for the very major operation which would be necessary.

Preoperative Preparation

The main problem concerns doing a major operation on a patient who is suffering from gross malnutrition. In comparatively early cases the operation can be done without special preparation but in severely malnourished patients some form of nutritional support is necessary to improve the patient's condition and so improve his chances of survival following a severe operation.

One way in which this can be done is to do a minor operation to introduce a feeding tube into the small intestine just beyond the duodenum. This is called a feeding jejunostomy. It is popular in parts of the world including Hong Kong but is rarely used in this country.

The two other alternatives are intravenous feeding or enteral feeding which is safe and inexpensive. The modern fine Clinifeed tubes can be passed into the stomach and left in place without complication and the patient is soon unaware of the tube.

Operations for Oesophageal Cancer

Apart from the major problem of correcting the nutritional defect it is necessary to have blood available for replacement during the operation and most surgeons will ask for an antibiotic cover. Different procedures are used for different levels of tumour. There is some argument among surgeons about the best operation for any particular case.

Lower Third Cancer of the Oesophagus

Access is usually by a left abdominothoracic incision but some thoracic surgeons do this operation through a left chest incision. An abdominothoracic incision extends from just above the umbilicus and crosses the costal margin so that the surgeon can excise about 8 inches of the 7th or 8th rib. Through this large incision the lower end of the oesophagus with the growth is excised with the spleen and the whole stomach. The intestinal continuity can be reconstructed in a number of ways but a popular technique is to use a piece of jejunum (Fig. 28).

Middle Third Cancer of the Oesophagus

It is impossible to reach the middle third of the oesophagus through the left chest but it is readily accessible through the right chest. Also it is not possible to use small intestine for the reconstruction as it will not reach high enough. Colon or stomach can be made to reach with ease. The operation therefore consists of a preliminary abdominal operation in which the stomach is fully mobilised so that it can be pulled up into the chest. The patient is then turned to his side and a second

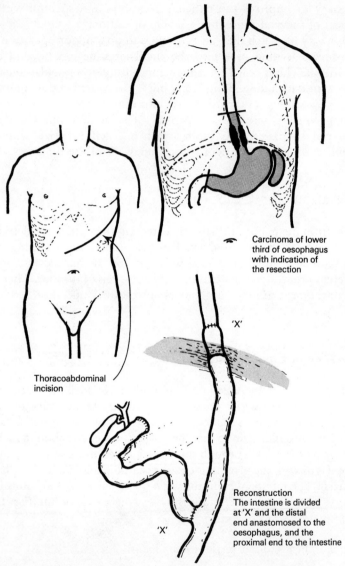

Carcinoma of lower
third of oesophagus
with indication of
the resection

Thoracoabdominal
incision

'X'

Reconstruction
The intestine is divided
at 'X' and the distal
end anastomosed to the
oesophagus, and the
proximal end to the intestine

'X'

Fig 28 Operation for carcinoma of the lower third of the oesophagus

operation done in which the right chest is opened by resecting about
half the 6th right rib. Through this incision the growth in the
oesophagus is mobilised and the stomach pulled up and joined to
the oesophagus where it has been divided above the growth
(Fig. 29).

Upper Third and Cervical Cancer of the Oesophagus

In this operation the two parts of the operation described for cancer of the middle third are completed. The chest is then closed and a third operation done in the neck. The oesophagus is identified. As the

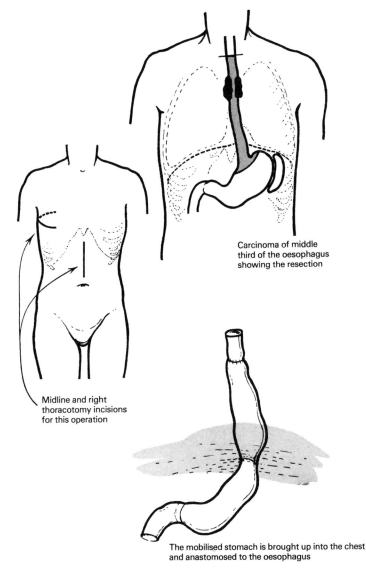

Carcinoma of middle
third of the oesophagus
showing the resection

Midline and right
thoracotomy incisions
for this operation

The mobilised stomach is brought up into the chest
and anastomosed to the oesophagus

Fig 29 Operation for carcinoma of middle third of oesophagus

oesophagus and stomach have been fully mobilised the stomach can be pulled up through this incision and sutured to the cut end of the oesophagus above the growth. The stomach readily reaches this level. Some surgeons prefer to use the colon but the operation is even longer and more complicated.

Postoperative Management

The patient will return from the operation to the ward with an intravenous infusion and also a 'gastric' tube, although in cases of total gastrectomy this tube will be in the jejunum. The surgeon will probably have passed the tube through the anastomosis and it is important to fix the tube well to the nostril so that it does not come up. If it does accidentally come up the nurse should not try to replace it without consulting the surgical staff as it is possible to damage the anastomosis and even cause a leak by reinserting the gastric tube.

Chest films are taken daily to assess the condition of the lungs and the pleural cavities which have been opened.

There will also be a thoracotomy tube in the chest which has been opened and this will be on closed drainage. Most surgeons remove the thoracotomy tube on the second or third day and take a further chest X-ray immediately after removal to see if any air was let into the pleura at the time of removal.

Oral fluids are usually limited to 30 ml hourly from the first day. Complete deprivation of oral fluid is unnecessary as there is up to 1 litre of saliva which has to pass the anastomosis and some water to wash this down can do no harm. The gastric tube passed through the anastomosis will drain off any surplus fluid which accumulates below the anastomosis. Oral fluids can be increased on about the third day and the patient should be on a light diet about the end of the week.

The main complication of oesophageal resection is leakage from the anastomosis. Should this happen the general condition of the patient will deteriorate and the X-ray will show fluid and air in the pleura or mediastinum. If leakage is suspected it can be confirmed by taking X-rays after giving the patient barium to drink.

Palliative Treatment

In many cases the tumour cannot be removed because of its attachment to other vital structures or it is pointless to remove because there are distant metastases in the liver or other places. In spite of this the patient needs treatment to enable him to swallow. In the

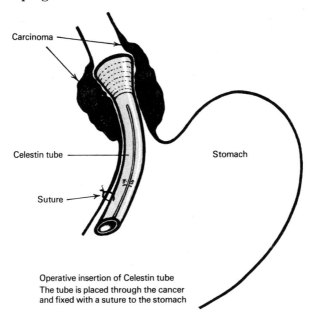

Carcinoma

Celestin tube

Suture

Stomach

Operative insertion of Celestin tube
The tube is placed through the cancer
and fixed with a suture to the stomach

Fig 30 Intubation for inoperable cancer of oesophagus

last stages when the oesophagus is completely obstructed even saliva which is swallowed is regurgitated and the patient literally drowns in his own saliva. To overcome this the tumour can be intubated. This means that a tube is placed within the growth so allowing food and drink to pass through the obstruction. Although the patient will still die from the growth he will not suffer so much from the problems of an obstructed oesophagus. Most of the tubes in use today are Celestin tubes. The modern tube is flexible and does not narrow when it is bent. It is made of latex rubber and strengthened with a spiral of nylon which can be seen in the substance of the latex. It has a funnel shape at the top which directs food into the tube and at the same time prevents the tube itself from slipping through the growth. It is also necessary to prevent the tube from coming up from its position in the growth into the throat. The tube which is placed at operation is sutured into the wall of the stomach and the tube which is placed through an endoscope has a reversed funnel at the lower end which prevents upward displacement.

Preoperative Preparation

There is no special preoperative preparation for endoscopic place-ment of a tube but if an operation is proposed it is sometimes necessary to improve the patient's nutrition before the operation. This can be done intravenously when it is called parenteral nutrition or by feeding the patient through a fine tube which can be passed through the growth into the stomach. This is called enteral feeding. Enteral feeding is safer and easier and the introduction of very fine plastic tubes such as the Clinifeed has made this technique popular.

Operative Intubation with a Celestin Tube

This is usually done when the patient has been explored for a resection but the growth has proved to be inoperable. The stomach is opened and a firm tube passed up the oesophagus and through the growth until it can be picked up by the anaesthetist. The anaesthetist attaches the Celestin tube and the surgeon is then able to haul it down until the funnel rests on top of the growth. The lower end of the tube is cut off in the stomach and it is attached to the wall of the stomach with a stitch (Fig. 30).

Endoscopic Intubation

This technique is preferred if the cancer is diagnosed as inoperable as it is easier for the patient.

A fibreoptic endoscope is passed down to the growth and used to thread a fine guide wire through the growth into the stomach. Its position can be confirmed by taking an X-ray. Once the guide wire is in position the endoscope is withdrawn and increasingly large dilators are threaded onto the guide wire and passed through the growth. When the growth is dilated sufficiently the guide wire is withdrawn and the gastroscope reintroduced to guide the Celestin tube through the growth (Fig. 31).

Postoperative Care

The main danger of all types of intubation is that the growth will be split by the dilatation with resulting leakage of oesophageal contents. This leakage takes place into the tissue surrounding the oesophagus which is called the mediastinum or into the pleural cavity. The oesophagus contains air and if a leak is present air can be seen on an X-ray in the mediastinum or in the pleural cavity where it is called a pneumothorax. The important postoperative investigation is a chest X-ray on the morning following the operation.

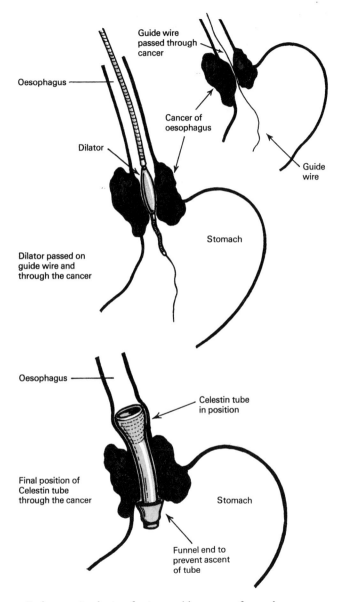

Fig 31 Endoscope intubation for inoperable cancer of oesophagus

The patient can be given food and drink after the operation provided there is no evidence of leakage from the oesophagus. Of course the latex tube is inert and food simply drops through into the stomach. The patient is told to take his meal slowly, to chew it well and to wash it down with plenty of fizzy drinks which help it through the tube. Large lumps of meat or vegetable will obviously block the tube which usually has a diameter of 12 mm. Given common sense and good advice the patient usually eats reasonably well and regains some weight.

Hiatus Hernia

A hiatus hernia is a herniation of part of the stomach through the opening in the diaphragm through which the oesophagus passes. There are two types. In one the fundus of the stomach herniates alongside the oesophagus but the oesophageal entry into the stomach is normal (Fig. 32). This is sometimes called a rolling hernia or a paraoesphageal hernia. In the second type the stomach and oeso-phagus slide up into the chest through the hiatus and the normal angle between the stomach and oesophagus is converted into a straight line (Fig. 33). This is called a sliding hiatus hernia. The first type is symptomless but may twist and cause a sudden surgical emergency. The second type is far more common and because the normal anatomy of the oesophagogastric angle is altered it is possible for gastric contents to reflux into the oesophagus. This reflux is the cause of all the symptoms and complications of sliding hiatus hernia.

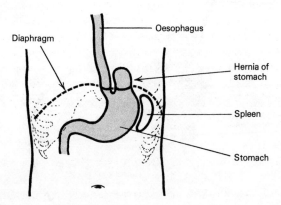

Fig 32   Paraoesophageal hiatus hernia

When gastric contents reflux into the oesophagus the lining is burned causing a condition called oesophagitis. The patient feels gastric contents in the throat as a burning sensation which is called heartburn. The patient with a sliding hiatus hernia tends to reflux more when stooping or lying down in bed as in the erect posture gravity prevents reflux.

When there is oesophagitis the patient often feels burning pain on swallowing and the pain may also be a constant one in the back or behind the sternum. The doctor may even diagnose angina because of severe retrosternal pain caused by oesophagitis. When the oesophagitis is severe and continues for a long time the inflammation in the lining of the oesophagus may begin to fibrose and eventually cause a stricture or narrowing so that the patient complains of increasing difficulty with swallowing his food. This symptom resembles the dysphagia seen in cancer of the oesophagus but the history is much longer. Another complication of reflux is inhalation of gastric contents causing inflammation in the lungs (pneumonitis). This often occurs at night when the patient is flat and fits of coughing at night may be caused by inhalation of refluxed gastric contents.

Diagnosis

In a clinically suspected case the diagnosis can be confirmed with a barium meal. During this examination the hernia is seen but the important part of the examination is the demonstration of reflux. With barium in the stomach the X-ray table can be tilted head down to encourage reflux. This does not occur in any position in a normal patient but can be demonstrated in most patients with a sliding hiatus hernia. Oesophagitis is better diagnosed by endoscopy when the fibreoptic oesophagoscope is passed under light sedation. The lining of the oesophagus is normally a very pale pink almost white colour but in oesophagitis it is seen to be bright red and it often bleeds on passage of the endoscope. A stricture of the oesophagus can be seen on both X-ray and oesophagoscopy.

Medical Treatment of Hiatus Hernia with Reflux Oesophagitis

Many patients with reflux are overweight and a programme of weight reduction is always helpful. Attempts to prevent reflux are difficult. Patients are often advised to sleep with blocks under the head of the bed and this may prevent some reflux. Advice to sleep in a sitting position in bed propped up with pillows is rarely successful and the patient finds himself flat by morning.

Drug treatment is sometimes successful in relieving oesophagitis but it cannot have any effect on reflux. Antacids have been used to neutralise gastric acid. More recently cimetidine has been used to reduce gastric acid secretion and so reduce the effects of acid oesophagitis. In some cases the oesophagitis is caused by bile reflux and these are not helped by cimetidine. Pyrogastrone is a drug which has been used with some success in acid and bile oesophagitis. This is a tablet containing antacid and carbenoxolone, which is used in the treatment of peptic ulcer, and alginic acid which gels in the stomach and converts the gastric contents to a jelly consistency, making reflux more difficult.

Surgical Treatment

The surgical correction of hiatus hernia and prevention of reflux is a difficult operation and is restricted to patients with severe oesophagitis who are reasonable operation risks.

The operation is approached in a variety of ways. It may be done through an abdominal or thoracic incision. Some surgeons find an abdominothoracic incision gives the best access. The operation is designed to reduce the hernia and to recreate the normal angle between the oesophagus and the stomach which prevents reflux. The hiatus is reduced in size leaving the oesophagus neatly fitting in the opening (Fig. 33). Another operation is called Nissen's fundoplication. The fundus of the stomach is wrapped round the oesophagus to produce a shape like an old fashioned inkwell.

Stricture of the Oesophagus

When a stricture of the oesophagus complicates longstanding oesophagitis the patient's nutrition is interfered with and some form of treatment is needed. In most cases it is possible to dilate the stricture with Eder–Puestow dilators through an endoscope (Fig. 31) and if the stricture recurs dilatation may be repeated. Dilatation combined with cimetidine has almost completely replaced the old operation in which the stricture was excised and replaced with a piece of colon.

Achalasia of the Cardia

Achalasia is an abnormality of the oesophagus which causes difficulty in swallowing (dysphagia). It is now thought that there is degeneration of the nerve fibres to the muscle of the oesophagus which results

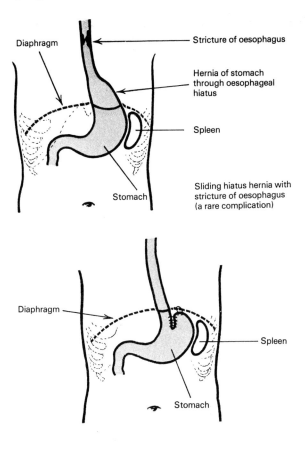

Diaphragm

Stricture of oesophagus

Hernia of stomach through oesophageal hiatus

Spleen

Stomach

Sliding hiatus hernia with stricture of oesophagus (a rare complication)

Diaphragm

Spleen

Stomach

Repair of sliding hiatus hernia
After reducing the hernia into the abdomen and reducing the size of the hiatus, the stomach is sutured to the oesophagus so restoring the normal angle between the stomach and oesophagus

Fig 33 Operation for hiatus hernia

in weak and uncoordinated peristalsis. As a result food passes slowly down the gullet, stops at the lower end and does not immediately enter the stomach. The abnormality is rare. It is most common between the ages of 30 and 50 years but may occur at any age.

Dysphagia is the presenting clinical symptom and is very slowly progressive. However, it does not often lead to wasting as the food eventually enters the stomach. When the oesophagus fills with food and drink it tends to regurgitate and patients with this condition rarely eat at restaurants because of the embarrassment caused by sudden regurgitation of the meal. Regurgitation at night may result in inhalation of food into the trachea and inflammation of the lungs (pneumonitis).

The diagnosis is confirmed by a barium swallow X-ray which shows the typical appearance.

Treatment

Treatment is by an operation which is called Heller's operation after its inventor. In this operation (Fig. 34) a longitudinal incision is made in the muscle of the oesophagus, and this allows the food to pass through easily. Most surgeons use a chest incision but some do the operation through the abdomen. The patient should be kept on fluids for some days prior to the operation so that there is no solid in the oesophagus and a gastric tube is passed into the oesophagus to aspirate fluid.

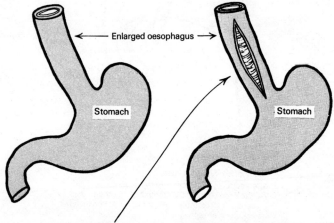

Enlarged oesophagus

Stomach

Stomach

Longitudinal incision in the thickened muscle coat of the oesophagus
The lining or mucosa of the oesophagus is left intact and is seen through the muscle split

Fig 34   Heller's operation for achalasia of the cardia

Postoperative Care

The patient is allowed fluid as soon as he wishes and food in 24 hours. The postoperative care is that of an ordinary thoracotomy with a thoracotomy drain.

Complications

The initial results of Heller's operation are excellent but there is a tendency for dysphagia to recur after many years. There is also a predisposition to cancer of the oesophagus.

15

Stomach and Duodenum

Anatomy and Physiology

Food passes through the gullet to reach the stomach which lies just below the diaphragm in the upper part of the abdomen. The stomach is the widest part of the alimentary canal and is capable of considerable enlargement to accommodate a large meal. A ring of muscle, called the pylorus, at the far end can close the outlet of the stomach so that the meal is retained there for a time during primary digestion and sterilisation by gastric acid. When the pyloric ring relaxes food passes into the next part of the alimentary canal which is called the duodenum. This is 'C' shaped with the head of the pancreas within the curve of the 'C' and with the bile and pancreatic ducts opening into its concavity (Fig. 17). The muscle of the stomach contracts in waves (a process called peristalsis) which pass from the oesophageal end to the pylorus so mixing and churning up the food with the various juices secreted by the stomach.

The stomach lining or mucosa is pitted with tiny openings which are the orifices of the gastric glands. These open onto the mucosa and are lined with cells which secrete enzymes and acid.

The stomach is divided into four parts which are the cardia, fundus, body and antrum (Fig. 35). These are physiological divisions and are based on the functions of these different parts of the stomach. There is no external sign of these differences and when the stomach is opened it is impossible to distinguish one part from another.

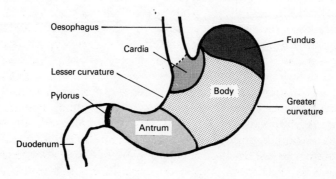

Fig 35 Anatomy of the stomach

The cardia is the part immediately adjacent to the point at which the oesophagus enters the stomach. The glands in this area secrete mucus which lubricates the passage of food and also protects the stomach wall from acid which is secreted from the body of the stomach.

The body and fundus of the stomach contain glands which are lined by three different types of secretory cells:

1   Parietal cells which secrete hydrochloric acid and a substance called intrinsic factor. One of the most important functions of gastric acid is to sterilise the food and prevent infection entering the body by this route, although it is obviously not always successful. In addition gastric acid provides a medium in which the enzyme pepsin is most active.

2   Chief cells secrete an enzyme called pepsin which begins the digestion of protein.

3   There are mucus secreting cells throughout the whole of the stomach.

The antrum of the stomach is completely different in function although identical in appearance. Again there are mucus secreting cells but instead of acid, the antrum secretes the alkali bicarbonate. In addition there are G cells which secrete a hormone, gastrin, which passes into the blood stream.

The duodenum also secretes bicarbonate which further neutralises gastric acid and provides a suitable environment for the function of the pancreatic enzymes which are delivered into the duodenum.

Regulation of Gastric Secretion

Gastric secretion is promoted by the sight and smell of food so that acid and enzymes are already appearing inside the stomach when food enters it from the oesophagus. This is called appetite juice. The sight and smell of food cause nerve impulses to go to the brain. Here the messages are diverted to a part of the brain called the hypothalamus and from here impulses go out through the vagus nerves which have branches to the stomach. One effect is to make the stomach contract causing peristaltic waves. Another is to cause the production of a chemical substance called histamine at the nerve endings. Histamine acts on a receptor called H_2 and this mediates in the production of gastric acid from the parietal or acid producing cells. It follows that if the vagus nerves are divided at an operation, gastric acid produced through this mechanism will cease. The drugs cimetidine and ranitidine prevent histamine acting on the H_2 receptor and have the same effect as vagotomy. If cimetidine does not reduce gastric acid in a particular case it is unlikely that the operation of vagotomy will reduce gastric acid as it works in a similar way (see p. 127).

A second phase of gastric secretion begins when food enters the stomach. Possibly as a result of distension of the antrum the G cells secrete the hormone gastrin directly into the blood stream. When blood containing gastrin reaches the gastric glands there is further secretion of acid and pepsin.

Investigations of the Stomach and Duodenum

1   Barium Meal

The most common investigation is the barium meal. Barium is the contrast material and the patient is screened in the X-ray department so that the radiologist can watch the barium filling the stomach. This examination is used when ulcer or cancer is suspected and a positive result will be obtained in a high percentage of cases. The patient must take nothing to eat or drink for six hours before the examination as food residue in the stomach interferes with the examination. It is wise to give an aperient after the examination as barium becomes very hard if it remains long in the colon.

2   Endoscopy

The fibreoptic gastroduodenoscope is passed under sedation and a view of the stomach and duodenum can be obtained. There is no permanent record other than the report of the operator. The advantages are that if a lesion is seen a biopsy can be taken for microscopic examination; also the lesion can be stroked with a brush and the material on the brush can be examined for cancer cells (cytology). The patient must be fasting for at least six hours to ensure the stomach is empty for the examination. Before passing the endoscope an anaesthetic lozenge is given or the pharynx is sprayed with a lignocaine anaesthetic spray. The throat will remain anaesthetised for some hours and it is important not to allow any food or drink for four hours after the examination. While the throat is anaesthetised there is a risk that anything taken by mouth may enter the trachea.

Many surgeons sedate patients with diazepam (Valium) and

because the effects may not pass off for many hours the patient must be told that it is dangerous to drive a car until the following day.

3   Insulin Test Meal

Most forms of test meal are now obsolete and will not be seen except during research projects. One exception to this is the insulin test meal which is used as a test of completeness of vagotomy. Insulin causes the level of sugar in the blood to be reduced (hypoglycaemia). If the blood sugar level reaches 35 mg % or lower the vagal nerves are stimulated and gastric acid is secreted. If the patient has had a vagotomy this cannot happen. If gastric acid is secreted this is evidence that the vagotomy was not complete.

The test is done by placing a gastric tube in the stomach. After giving 20 units of insulin the stomach is aspirated at 15 minute intervals for two hours and the specimens examined for acid. A patient who has had a vagotomy will not secrete more than 20 mmol/litre of acid in the two hours.

Symptoms of Gastroduodenal Diseases

Nausea is a feeling of sickness which may develop into vomiting. Vomiting is associated with many diseases of the stomach and duodenum, as well as some diseases outside the abdomen. When the pylorus is obstructed the vomit is large in volume and food which has remained in the stomach for 24 hours or more may be recognised by the patient. The act of vomiting is accompanied by sympathetic overactivity causing pallor and sweating and the glottis closes tightly to prevent the entry of vomit into the trachea. In an unconscious or partly conscious patient such as one recovering from an anaesthetic there is a risk that the glottis will not close so that vomit may be inhaled into the trachea. Inhalation of bile or acid gastric contents causes a serious inflammation in the lungs (inhalation pneumonitis) which may be fatal. An unconscious patient who vomits must be nursed lying on one side so encouraging the vomit to come out of the mouth. A sucker can be used to assist the removal of vomit from the mouth and back of the tongue.

Anorexia means loss of appetite and is a very marked symptom in cases of cancer of the stomach.

Heartburn is a burning sensation at the back of the tongue or in the throat. It is caused by the reflux of gastric contents up the oesophagus and is often a symptom of hiatus hernia when the normal valve mechanism at the gastro-oesophageal junction is not working.

Hiccough may be a symptom of renal failure (uraemia) but anything which presses on and irritates the diaphragm may cause spasmodic contractions of the diaphragm and typical hiccough. A distended stomach or colon, blood from injury to the spleen, or pus from a perforated ulcer are typical examples.

Pain is a common symptom of gastric or duodenal ulcer. It usually bears a constant relation to the taking of a meal. The pain of duodenal ulcer begins about two hours after a meal and wakes the patient at about 2 a.m. when the stomach is empty and free acid from the stomach runs over the ulcer. Pain is not a prominent feature of gastric cancer and this is one reason for the late presentation.

Peptic Ulceration

The most common sites for peptic ulcer are along the lesser curvature of the stomach (gastric ulcer) and in the first 2.5 cm of the duodenum (duodenal ulcer). Peptic ulceration has been diminishing in incidence in Britain during the past 30 years. The reason for this is unknown. During recent years there has been a further steep fall in the number of cases requiring surgical treatment because of the impact of the drugs cimetidine and ranitidine on the treatment of duodenal ulcer.

Chronic Gastric Ulcer

Gastric ulcer is much less common than duodenal ulcer and is now a rare disease. The sex incidence is about equal but duodenal ulcer is much more common in men. Gastric acidity is normal or low in cases of gastric ulcer and high in duodenal ulcer.

The diagnosis is suggested in a patient who has pain shortly after meals. It is confirmed by a barium meal and by endoscopy. There may be some difficulty in deciding if an ulcer is benign or malignant and this can be resolved by biopsy and cytology at the time of endoscopy.

Primary treatment is medical. If the patient is having severe symptoms a period of bed rest is advised but as soon as pain is relieved he may be ambulant.

It is important to avoid smoking and drugs which irritate the stomach such as aspirin and antirheumatic drugs like butazolidine and indomethecin.

Although doctors used to advise strict diets for patients with ulcers there is no evidence to support the use of any form of diet other than the avoidance of alcohol on an empty stomach and strongly spiced food.

A number of drugs are in use in the medical treatment of gastric ulcer:

Carbenoxolone (Biogastrone) has the disadvantage of causing sodium and water retention and should therefore be used with caution in patients with cardiac or renal complaints.

Caved-S is a preparation of liquorice which, it is claimed, does not cause any biochemical disturbance.

Bismuth components have been reintroduced in the form of chelated bismuth which is supposed to encourage healing by forming a protective layer over the ulcer.

Cimetidine is primarily used in the treatment of duodenal ulcer but has also been successfully used in the medical treatment of gastric ulcer.

In all cases being treated medically the effect of treatment is observed by further barium meal or endoscopy at intervals of four to six weeks until the ulcer is seen to be healed.

Surgical Treatment of Gastric Ulcer

If a gastric ulcer relapses after medical treatment the question of surgical treatment has to be discussed with the patient who will have to decide if an operation is preferred to the pain and other problems of a recurrent ulcer. Repeated periods away from work is often a factor influencing the patient to accept surgical treatment.

Surgical treatment is also necessary for the complications of a simple gastric ulcer. These are illustrated in Fig. 36 and comprise perforation, haemorrhage, stenosis and malignant change. The most popular operation is removal of about half the stomach including the ulcer and reconstruction by anastomosing the remaining part of the stomach to the duodenum (Billroth 1 gastrectomy – Fig. 42).

Chronic Duodenal Ulcer

Duodenal ulcer usually occurs in the first 2–3 cm of the duodenum. The most important factor in the aetiology of duodenal ulcer is an excess of acid secretion by the stomach. Smoking is also a factor and a stressful occupation may predispose to duodenal ulcer but many patients with duodenal ulcer come from humble backgrounds.

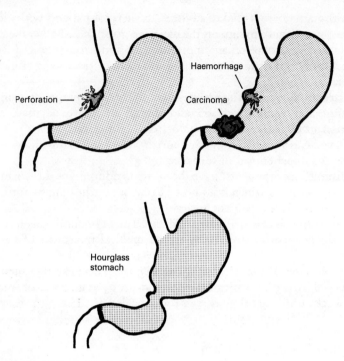

Fig 36 Complications of gastric ulcer

Diagnosis

The outstanding symptom of duodenal ulceration is pain which usually occurs 2–3 hours after a meal. Some patients find that the pain is relieved by a meal and another characteristic feature is that the pain wakes the patient around 2 or 3 a.m. in the night when it can be relieved by taking a drink of milk. Vomiting is an occasional feature. Patients who endure the pain of duodenal ulcer over a long period of time develop a characteristic drawn facial expression.

The diagnosis is confirmed by barium meal and by endoscopy.

Medical Treatment

The drugs cimetidine and ranitidine have had a very important impact on the treatment of duodenal ulcer and since their introduction the number of operations done for ulcer has dropped dramatically. Cimetidine acts by preventing the action of the vagus nerves on the acid secreting cells of the stomach. It is given in a dose of 200 mg three times daily with a dose of 400 mg last thing at night. The course is for six weeks and it is usual to maintain the night dose for up to three months. With this suppression of gastric acid secretions, most ulcers become asymptomatic in a few days. At the present time alkalis to neutralise acid and other drugs are rarely used. There is no need to impose any dietary restrictions but the patient is advised not to smoke.

Surgical Treatment

The operation for duodenal ulcer is division of the vagus nerves which stimulate the acid secreting (parietal) cells. This operation is called vagotomy (Fig. 37). One way of doing this operation is to divide the nerves where they are in large trunks above the stomach. This operation is called truncal vagotomy. The vagus nerves send branches to most of the abdominal viscera and all the intestine, and it is surprising that their division has no obvious effect on intestinal movement. Some surgeons do an operation in which the nerves are

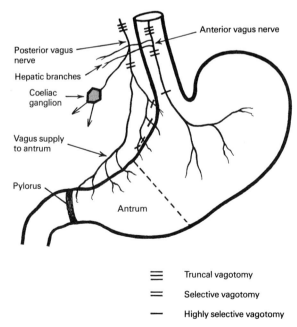

Fig 37   Types of vagotomy

divided a little lower down so that only the branches to the stomach are divided with preservation of the branches to the rest of the abdomen. This operation is called selective vagotomy. In addition to reducing gastric acid secretion vagotomy paralyses the stomach so that it does not empty easily into the duodenum. To overcome this problem an additional procedure is required. One operation is to divide the pylorus and make the exit from the stomach larger (pyloroplasty). Another way is to attach a loop of small intestine to the greater curve of the stomach to assist the emptying. This is called gastrojejunostomy because the stomach is joined to the small intestine which is called the jejunum (Fig. 38). There is a third form of

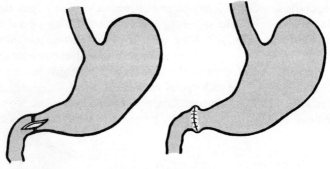

Pylorplasty
An incision is made across the pylorus and sutured in the opposite direction

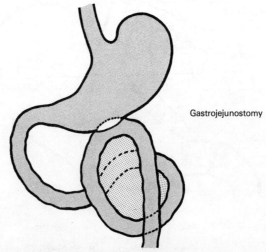

Gastrojejunostomy

A loop of small intestine is sutured to the greater curvature of the stomach

Fig 38   Gastric drainage operations

vagotomy which is called highly selective vagotomy in which the vagus nerves to the upper two-thirds of the stomach are divided so denervating the acid secreting cells. The vagus nerve to the antrum is left intact. The antrum does not have any acid secreting cells and because its vagus nerve supply is left intact it remains active and peristalsis takes the food and sends it through the pylorus into the duodenum. The advantage of this operation is that it is not necessary to do a drainage operation as the stomach empties normally.

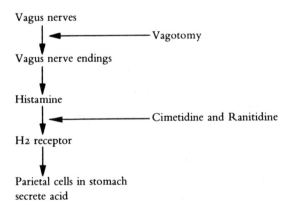

Highly selective vagotomy

This diagram illustrates the train of reaction between an impulse transmitted down the vagus nerve to the final result of secretion of acid and also the way in which surgical and medical treatment interfere with the effect of vagus nerve stimulation.

Vagus nerves ←————— Vagotomy

Vagus nerve endings

Histamine ←————— Cimetidine and Ranitidine

H2 receptor

Parietal cells in stomach secrete acid

In patients in whom the ulcer recurs after vagotomy the antrum may be removed. This results in further reduction of acid secretion by removing the gastrin mechanism.

Postoperative Management

Following vagotomy the patient will return to the ward with an intravenous infusion and a gastric tube which should be connected to a drainage bag. The intravenous fluid will be prescribed by the doctor and it is important to maintain the flow at the correct speed which will allow the infusion of the correct amount of fluid in the day. If there is a fault causing delay with the infusion this should be reported to the doctor. The details of oral fluid are also at the discretion of the doctor. After vagotomy there is temporary difficulty with emptying of the stomach caused by its paralysis and temporary swelling of the anastomosis. Highly selective vagotomy does not need a drainage operation and patients who have this operation usually recover more quickly. The gastric tube is left in the stomach and oral fluids are restricted to 30 ml hourly for the first 24 hours. When the aspirated fluid is less than the intake the oral fluid can be increased. Commonly the intake is increased to 60 ml hourly and the next day to unlimited fluid. At this stage, when the patient is taking fluid freely, the intravenous infusion can be discontinued. Patients should be out of bed on the day following operation and can easily sit in a chair with an intravenous infusion and gastric tube.

Complications of Peptic Ulcer (Figs. 36 and 39)

The complications of gastric and duodenal ulcers are so similar that they can be described together. There has been a dramatic fall in the number of hospital admissions for perforation and haemorrhage complicating chronic peptic ulcer which is almost certainly due to the effect of cimetidine in healing ulcers.

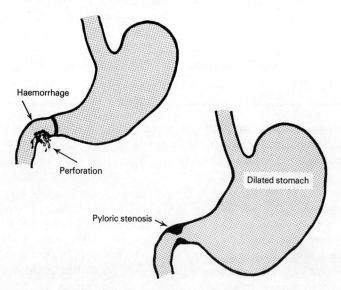

Fig 39   Complications of duodenal ulcer

Perforation

Perforation of a gastric or duodenal ulcer is one of the great emergencies of surgery. As the gastric or duodenal contents flood into the peritoneal cavity there is an immediate chemical inflammation of the peritoneal cavity caused by acid and bile. This causes severe pain which comes on with great suddenness coinciding with the perforation. The muscles of the abdomen become rigid like a board. If left untreated the peritoneal cavity becomes infected resulting in bacterial peritonitis. Without surgical treatment a fatal result is almost certain.

The operation consists of simple closure of the perforation. In some cases, particularly when the perforation is seen at an early stage and when the surgeon is experienced, a vagotomy may be done after the closure, to prevent recurrence of the ulcer.

The patient is prepared for surgery in the usual way. Probably an intravenous infusion will be set up in the ward and a gastric tube placed in the stomach, but this is sometimes done in the anaesthetic room or during the operation. Following the operation the regimen is the same as following vagotomy with the addition of antibiotics to control peritoneal infection.

Acute Haemorrhage

Sudden bleeding from a chronic peptic ulcer is usually due to the penetration of a large artery in the base of the ulcer. The patient's stomach and intestines fill with blood and he vomits blood (haematemesis). Blood which is vomited after a period of time in the stomach is partly digested and resembles coffee grounds. Blood passed from the rectum is called melaena. After passing through the intestine blood resembles tar with some brighter red patches. Such severe bleeding causes circulatory collapse (shock). The blood pressure falls and the pulse rate rises. The patient looks pale from constriction of the peripheral blood vessels and may faint because of diminished blood flow to the brain. There are a number of causes of acute gastroduodenal haemorrhage but the shock demands immediate treatment and precedes any detailed studies concerning the cause of the bleeding. The subject of shock is dealt with in more detail in Chapter 7. The essentiality is the replacement of blood lost in sufficient quantity to restore the circulation. Ten ml of blood are taken from a vein and placed in a sterile bottle for grouping and cross matching with donor blood and the estimated initial requirements are ordered from the blood bank.

While waiting for blood to arrive from the bank, an intravenous infusion is set up with dextrose saline or Hartmann's solution. These solutions are rapidly lost in the urine and it is better to change to something which will remain in the circulation and so maintain the blood pressure for a longer period. Dextran and plasma can be used but the product called Haemaccel, which is gelatin with added sodium, potassium, calcium and chloride is safer and has the additional advantage of being inexpensive (at the time of writing 500 ml costs less than £2). When blood arrives from the bank it is used in place of the Haemaccel.

A central venous catheter is put in position and measurement of the central venous pressure is used to determine the amount of blood transfusion required. Too much blood can overload the circulation and cause heart failure and a raised central venous pressure. Too little does not relieve the shock. The central venous pressure is kept as near to normal as possible by regulating the volume of transfusion. There is no set rate for transfusion but the amount given is that required to correct the shock and depends mainly on the amount lost.

A catheter is put into the bladder so that the output of urine can be measured.

The nurse has many responsibilities in cases of acute haemorrhage. The blood pressure, pulse rate and central venous pressure are measured at 15 minute intervals as they reflect the state of shock. The volume of intravenous fluid and the volume of catheter drainage have to be charted. A gastric tube is usually put into the stomach but blood in the stomach clots and cannot be aspirated.

Diagnosis.   The exact cause of the bleeding may be judged from the history and clinical signs. For example the patient may be known to have a chronic gastric or duodenal ulcer.

Another cause of acute bleeding is an acute ulcer or ulcers. When an ulcer is confined to the mucosa of the stomach it is called an erosion and those penetrating into the muscle are called acute ulcers. Both may be multiple in the acute phase and both may present with serious bleeding. These patients usually have no preceding history or a short period of two or three days dyspepsia. Acute ulcers or erosions may be caused by aspirin or antirheumatic drugs such as indomethecin. Often these drugs have been taken by mouth but there is also a systemic effect as indomethecin given by suppository may also cause acute gastric ulcers.

In the condition of portal hypertension, which often complicates liver cirrhosis, the pressure in the veins leading to the liver is raised because of obstruction in the liver. This results in varicose dilatation of the veins and those in the stomach and oesophagus bulge through the mucosa and may burst causing serious bleeding. However, bleeding in patients with varices may not be from the varices but from acute erosions or ulcers in the stomach which sometimes complicate this condition.

Barium meal examination and endoscopy using a fibreoptic gastroduodenoscope are often used in difficult cases. Endoscopy is more informative as shallow ulcers are not seen with X-rays. An important part of endoscopy is that the examination is done on a patient with an empty stomach but in acute haemorrhage the stomach is filled with blood and clot which prevents a clear view. Following endoscopy the patient needs special nursing care. The throat is partly anaesthetised to assist the passage of the endoscope and this effect may be expected to last for up to three hours following return to the ward. Vomiting of blood during this time is very dangerous as it may be inhaled into the trachea. The patient is nursed on the side and after vomiting the sucker is used to aspirate blood from the back of the mouth and throat to minimise the risk of inhalation.

Surgical Treatment. In most cases haemorrhage from a chronic duodenal ulcer stops naturally but if it continues and particularly if the patient is elderly or there is difficulty with blood transfusion an operation may be advised to stop the bleeding. In developing countries where blood transfusion facilities are limited it is necessary to operate more often and at an earlier stage to conserve blood.

At the operation the stomach or duodenum is opened to expose the ulcer. Usually the bleeding artery can be seen and a suture is run under it to stop the flow of blood. In addition a vagotomy is done, but if the patient is too ill for this he can be given cimetidine to reduce the acid.

Pyloric Stenosis

Longstanding duodenal ulceration may result in excessive scarring which narrows and partly obstructs the passage of food through the pylorus. The stomach enlarges and its muscle coat becomes thicker and stronger so that peristalsis tries to push food through the narrow pylorus. The diagnosis is suggested by a history of ulcer with recent increasing vomiting. The vomit is particularly copius and may contain food taken more than 24 hours earlier. Examination shows a patient who has lost weight and locally the outline of the stomach can be seen with visible peristalsis. This means that when the upper part of the abdomen is inspected the stomach contractions are so strong that they can be seen through the abdominal wall.

The diagnosis can be confirmed by doing a barium meal which shows food residue in the stomach and delay in emptying of a very large stomach.

The vomiting of pyloric stenosis causes complicated biochemical changes. Repeated vomiting leads to loss of food and water so that patients lose weight and become dehydrated. The stomach normally produces hydrochloric acid (HCl) which is a strong acid. If the pyloric sphincter is open the loss of stomach acid is neutralised by the loss of bicarbonate which is secreted in the duodenum and also vomited. In pyloric stenosis the vomiting results in loss of acid alone and the body becomes relatively alkaline. This is called alkalosis. There is also loss of chloride which causes a low blood chloride (hypochloraemia). A further complication of alkalosis is that potassium (K) is lost in excess in the urine resulting in a low blood potassium (hypokalaemia). The loss of fluid also results in a rise in the blood urea due to the dehydration and not to any abnormality of the kidney, a condition sometimes called extrarenal uraemia.

So in pyloric stenosis the biochemical changes are:

1   dehydration resulting in mild uraemia;
2   alkalosis;
3   hypokalaemia (low K) and hypochloraemia (low Cl). The other electrolytes in the blood are normal.

Treatment of Pyloric Stenosis

The surgical treatment of pyloric stenosis is pyloroplasty or gastrojejunostomy and these operations are illustrated in Fig. 38. In addition a vagotomy should be performed to reduce acid production by the stomach and prevent recurrent ulceration.

Before embarking on surgery the patient must be prepared. This consists of two parts:

1   correction of the biochemical disorder by giving intravenous 0.9 % isotonic sodium chloride with added potassium;
2   the dilated stomach presents technical difficulties to the surgeon and a gastric tube is left in the stomach for two or three days of preparation.

In some cases with an excessive food residue a large gastric tube is passed to get rid of the excess of food which will not come up through the usual small bore tube. The patient is restricted to liquid feeding which will pass through the narrow pylorus.

Tumours of the Stomach

Nearly all tumours of the stomach are malignant adenocarcinomas. Benign tumours are occasionally seen. These may be adenoma, a benign tumour arising from the cells of the mucosa, or leiomyoma, a tumour arising from the muscle of the stomach wall. Among malignant tumours there is the malignant form of the muscle tumour which is called a leiomyosarcoma and lymphoma which is a tumour of the lymphatic tissue of the stomach.

Carcinoma of the Stomach

Gastric carcinoma is a very serious form of cancer with a high mortality even after surgical excision. The disease is rare in Africa. In Europe and the United States it is becoming less common and it is estimated that there has been a 30 % decrease in incidence during the last 30 years. On the other hand, in parts of Southern Russia and in Japan there has been a dramatic increase in gastric cancer. Japanese living in the USA have a risk of gastric cancer identical with indigenous Americans so that the causative factor is not race. Dietary factors have been suggested but not proved.

Patients who do not secrete acid in the stomach (achlorhydria) have a high risk of developing gastric cancer. One example of this is the disease known as pernicious anaemia which is characterised by achlorhydria. In this disease there is a high incidence of gastric cancer and about 6 % of patients with pernicious anaemia die from carcinoma of the stomach. Indigestion developing in a patient with pernicious anaemia should be investigated at once.

It has been noted that patients of blood group A have a higher incidence of stomach cancer.

Types of Gastric Cancer (Fig. 40)

1 **Mucosal carcinoma** is asymptomatic and can only be diagnosed by endoscopy. There is a small area of abnormal appearance in which the cells have the appearance under the microscope of cancer cells but there is no infiltration into the deeper

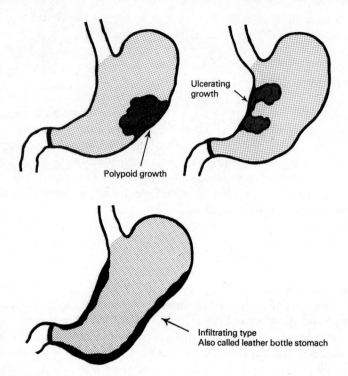

Fig 40 Types of gastric cancer

layer. This is a form of 'cancer *in situ*' in which the cells have become malignant but have not migrated from their normal site. This type of gastric cancer has only been recognised since the introduction of gastroscopy. In Japan, where there is a great awareness of the danger of gastric cancer, there are programmes of routine endoscopy of asymptomatic patients and this has led to the identification of mucosal cancer. In this country where the disease is rare and decreasing in incidence mucosal lesions are not often found.

2 In **polypoid cancer** the tumour forms a large mass projecting into the lumen of the stomach.

3 **Ulcerating cancer** is a type in which the centre of the tumour sloughs out to leave a large ulcer.

4 **Infiltrating cancer** is a type in which the tumour spreads through the wall of the stomach converting it into a rigid bag. This is sometimes called a leather bottle stomach.

5 **Ulcer cancer** must be distinguished from ulcerating cancer, which is a term to describe a particular type of appearance. The term ulcer cancer implies that the cancer has arisen in a previously existing benign gastric ulcer. Malignant change in a benign ulcer is very rare.

Spread

Local spread is to the adjacent organs. In particular this may lead to involvement of the colon, pancreas, liver and to important blood vessels. Such local spread may render the tumour irremovable.

Lymphatic spread is mainly to the lymph nodes around the stomach. Cancer cells may also enter the main lymph duct in the abdomen behind the stomach and be carried up into the neck to involve the lymph nodes above the clavicle. Enlargement of the supraclavicular lymph nodes by cancer of the stomach has been known for a very long time and is called Troisier's sign. Biopsy or aspiration cytology of such a node may give the diagnosis.

Blood stream spread takes place when cancer cells enter the veins of the stomach. These veins carry blood to the liver where cancer cells are filtered off and multiply to form metastases.

Cells may also separate from the main mass in the stomach and drop off into the peritoneal cavity. The multiplication of these cells results in small metastatic tumours throughout the peritoneal cavity. The resulting inflammation of the peritoneum causes an exudate of fluid which gradually fills the abdominal cavity. This is called ascites. If cells reach and get implanted onto the surface of an ovary they may grow into a very large ovarian tumour.

Diagnosis

If the carcinoma arises near the cardia of the stomach it will result in difficulty in swallowing (dysphagia) at an early stage. A tumour at the pylorus causes early pyloric obstruction with symptoms of vomiting of food (Fig. 41). Many tumours arise in the body of the stomach and remain silent for a long time. As the tumour enlarges in the stomach the patient complains of severe loss of appetite (anorexia) and loses weight. The tumour usually bleeds slowly into the stomach and the patient gradually becomes anaemic from blood loss. The presenting symptoms may result from the anaemia. For example, the patient may complain of pallor or shortness of breath. Symptoms related to the stomach are not usually marked and are more like a dyspepsia than an ulcer. Severe pain after meals suggests a benign ulcer. Vomiting blood is also usually a sign of a benign ulcer although a gastric cancer may occasionally bleed seriously.

Investigations

The first investigation is usually a barium meal examination which shows the cancer bulging into the stomach. Endoscopy is also used

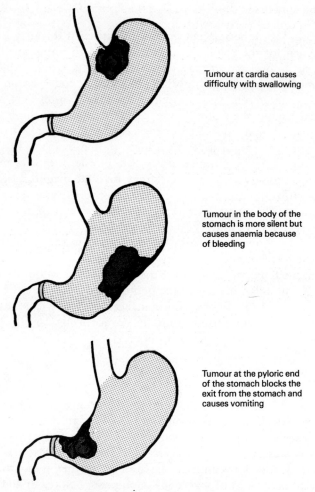

Tumour at cardia causes difficulty with swallowing

Tumour in the body of the stomach is more silent but causes anaemia because of bleeding

Tumour at the pyloric end of the stomach blocks the exit from the stomach and causes vomiting

Fig 41 Symptoms of cancer of the stomach

and has the advantage that small pieces can be taken for histological examination so confirming the diagnosis. This is especially important when there is doubt about the possible malignant character of an ulcer in the stomach.

Treatment

Carcinoma of the stomach is resistant to all forms of radiation and chemotherapy and the only hope of cure is surgical removal. If the tumour is situated in the distal half of the stomach it is usually treated by an adequate partial gastrectomy (Fig. 42). More extensive tumours and those involving the proximal part of the stomach are treated by total gastrectomy. In some cases the surgeon will remove adjacent organs which are infiltrated by the growth. These include part of the pancreas, the spleen, and transverse colon. There is a variety of ways of reconstructing the anatomy but a common operation is the use of a piece of intestine introduced by a technique called a Roux loop. Access to the stomach for these operations is usually through an upper abdominal incision, but if the surgeon intends to do a total gastrectomy the incision may be abdomino-thoracic (Fig. 28). If the surgeon finds that he is unable to remove the tumour it may be possible to do a palliative operation. This is an operation which makes the symptoms less troublesome and the remaining life of the patient more tolerable although the tumour is not removed. An example of this is a gastrojejunostomy which may relieve symptoms of pyloric obstruction (Fig. 38).

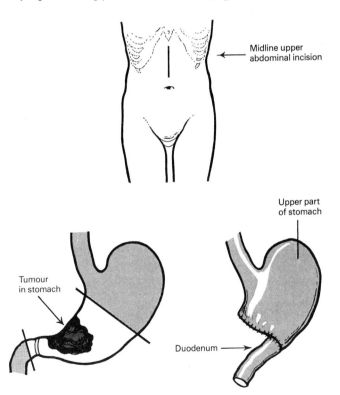

Fig 42 Partial gastrectomy for cancer of the stomach

Preoperative Preparation

The tests done before the operation will include electrolytes, liver
function tests and blood count. If the patient is anaemic he will be
transfused and any electrolyte abnormality which might result from
vomiting is corrected by intravenous therapy.

Many patients have chronic chest troubles and routine breathing
exercises are started before the operation. Some surgeons like to give
an antibiotic cover to the operation.

Postoperative Management

A gastric tube is passed by the anaesthetist during some stage of the
operation. When the patient returns to the ward following the
operation he will have an indwelling gastric tube, an intravenous drip
infusion, and possibly a tube drain. If the operation has been done
through an abdominothoracic approach there will also be a thoracotomy drain. All of these tubes need special care which is described
in Chapters 4 and 22.

Oral fluids are limited to 30 ml hourly in the first 24 hours. There is
always some swelling at the suture lines and fluid which is taken by
mouth cannot pass out into the intestine until this swelling subsides.
Complete deprivation of fluid is very unpleasant for the patient and
the small amount given by mouth will return through the gastric tube
if it accumulates in the stomach remnant. Oral fluids are increased
daily, usually to 60 ml and then to 90 ml hourly before going to free
fluids on about the third or fourth day. After this a light diet is
introduced. If the amount of fluid aspirated from the gastric tube
remains high, possibly in excess of the fluid taken, this programme has
to be slowed down and the patient kept on 30 ml or 60 ml hourly
until the aspirate is reduced. There is very little risk of breakdown of
the suture line following a partial gastrectomy but there is a real risk
after total gastrectomy. The oesophagus is notorious for its difficulty
in healing and the introduction of a light diet is usually delayed until
about the seventh day. Also in total gastrectomy the 'gastric' tube is
introduced into the intestine below the anastomosis by the surgeon at
the time of the operation. It is most important that this tube should
not be accidentally withdrawn as its reintroduction through the
anastomosis may be very dangerous as it is possible to pass the tube
through the suture line, thus making a hole through which oral fluid
will leak.

16

Small Intestine

Anatomy and Physiology

The small intestine is a tube about 6 metres long which extends from the duodenum to the colon, which it joins at the caecum. It is divided into jejunum, which is the first part, and ileum, which is the second half. There is no exact point at which the intestine changes from one to the other and in fact there is very little difference in the appearance of the intestine from one end to the other but the proximal part is somewhat thicker and the distal part thinner and almost transparent.

The intestine is a muscular tube and peristaltic contractions move the food contents along its length. The inner lining of the intestine is called the mucosa. This is not a simple flat surface because this would not afford a sufficient surface area for all the food digestion and absorption. There are folds of mucosa which can easily be seen, but the main increase in surface area is caused by little projections which can be seen with a low power microscope and are called villi. In between the villi there are tiny pits which are called glands or crypts (Crypts of Lieberkuhn) (Fig. 43). The whole area is covered with columnar-shaped cells. Those in the bottom of the crypts are among the most rapidly dividing cells in the body and the new cells grow up towards the surface where they are shed from the mucosa into the lumen of the intestine. These cells, which have a life of only two or three days, are digested in the intestine and reabsorbed, so forming a cycle of protein metabolism within the body and conserving it for re-use. The cells which cover the villi are also covered with tiny microvilli which can be seen only with the electron microscope and this still further increases the functional area of the intestine. Eight to ten litres of fluid with 1500 mmol of sodium and 100 mmol of potassium pass into the intestine daily. Virtually all is reabsorbed for re-use.

Carbohydrates such as glucose are absorbed into the blood stream by simple diffusion.

Proteins are first broken down into peptides by the enzyme trypsin which is produced by the pancreas. The final digestion into the amino acids, which are the building blocks of proteins, is brought about by enzymes which are secreted in the microvilli. Amino acids are

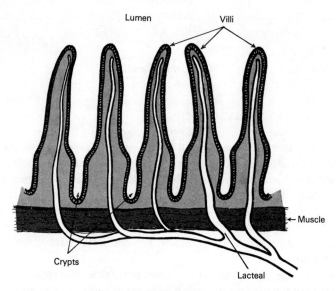

Fig 43   Magnification of wall of small intestine

absorbed into the blood stream and carried to the liver.

Fats are not water soluble and cannot be absorbed in this simple way. They are first digested by pancreatic lipase which converts fat into fatty acids and monoglycerides which are also insoluble in water. However the bile salts have a detergent effect on the products of fat digestion and convert them into tiny particles called micelles which are absorbed into the villi. Once in the cells of the villi the micelles join together to form larger particles which are discharged into a lymph duct or lacteal which exists in the centre of each villus. Once in the lymph duct the fat particles move along lymph vessels in the mesentery. The mesenteric lymph vessels join the main lymph duct which passes up through the back of the chest and finally joins the great veins in the neck where recently eaten and digested fat reaches the blood stream in the form of tiny fat particles (Fig. 97).

Most digestion and absorption takes place in the upper half of the intestine and there is a great deal of spare capacity. Considerable lengths of intestine can be removed without interfering with nutrition. However, the distal intestine is especially important for the absorption of vitamin B12 and bile salts which are absorbed and recirculated. Excision of the terminal ileum may result in loss of these substances.

Crohn's Disease

This disease was first described in 1932 by Crohn, an American physician. It may affect any part of the intestine but characteristically the disease begins and is most severe in the terminal ileum. Sometimes other parts of the intestine are affected with normal intervening segments called 'skip' areas. The cause is unknown. The bowel wall thickens and the mucosal lining is greatly deformed and has the appearance of cobblestones. Abscesses may form alongside the intestine and these may rupture causing a sinus to the skin or a fistulous connection between the terminal ileum and another piece of intestine.

Symptoms

In the early stages Crohn's disease of the intestine is silent and the clinical presentation is caused by the complications.

The narrow segment of intestine may cause chronic intestinal obstruction and the patient complains of intermittent colicky abdominal pain sometimes accompanied by loud intestinal sounds as the excessive peristalsis tries to overcome the partial obstruction. Many patients complain of diarrhoea.

In severe cases an abscess may form in the right iliac fossa and the patient may be operated on as an acute appendicitis. Some cases present with complex anal fistulae which do not respond to the usual treatment.

Disease in the terminal ileum prevents the resorption of bile salts which are lost in the faeces. As bile salts hold cholesterol in solution in bile, disease or removal of the terminal ileum may be complicated by cholesterol gallstones.

In cases which have had some intestine removed and also have extensive recurrent disease there are severe nutritional problems because of malabsorption by the diseased intestinal mucosa. The diagnosis can be confirmed by barium meal or enema.

Treatment

Recurrence following surgical removal of intestine for Crohn's disease is so common that surgeons now avoid resection unless there are complications.

Medical treatment comprises general measures such as treatment of anaemia and defective nutrition. In many cases this is all that is necessary but in the acute phase steroid therapy is often used. Although the cause of Crohn's disease is unknown some authorities have suggested that it is an autoimmune disease and this is the basis of treatment with the immuno-suppressive drug azathioprine.

Surgical treatment is usually advised for complications. The most common complication requiring surgery is chronic intestinal obstruction. The intestine may be removed if the affected segment is short but when there is extensive disease it is better not to sacrifice any intestine and to do a short-circuit operation (Fig. 44).

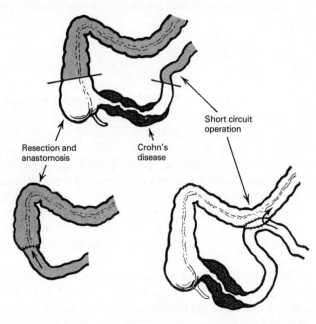

Fig 44 Surgical treatment of Crohn's disease of ileum

Tumours of the Small Intestine

Tumours of the small intestine are rare while tumours of the large intestine are common.

Benign tumours such as adenoma and lipoma are occasionally seen. Among malignant tumours, the reticulum cell sarcoma arising in the lymphatic tissue and adenocarcinoma arising from the glandular mucosa are the most common.

Carcinoid Tumour

One remarkable tumour of the small intestine arises from cells in the mucosa which are called argentaffin cells because they have an affinity for silver stains when stained in the laboratory. In the appendix the carcinoid tumour (sometimes called an argentaffinoma) is usually benign and an incidental finding in appendicectomy. However, when it occurs in the small intestine it is usually malignant though patients often live for many years and malignancy is low. The interest lies in the fact that the cells produce a hormone called 5-hydroxytryptamine (5-HT) which produces dramatic symptoms. These comprise attacks of flushing of the face, diarrhoea, and asthmatic attacks. The tumour metastasises to the liver and the hormone effects are usually seen when liver metastases are present. The diagnosis is confirmed by the identification of 5-hydroxyindoleacetic acid (5-HIAA), which is a product of 5-HT, in the urine. This is called the carcinoid syndrome.

Treatment

Benign tumours of the small intestine are removed if they are diagnosed but malignant tumours are rarely removable. If they are causing intestinal obstruction this can be relieved by doing a short-circuit operation.

Obstruction of the Small Intestine

Obstruction of the small intestine may occur as a sudden, dramatic incidence when it is called acute intestinal obstruction. In some cases there is interference with the blood supply to the intestine as well as blockage of the lumen. This is called a strangulated obstruction and is a more serious type of intestinal obstruction. All forms of acute intestinal obstruction demand immediate surgical treatment if the patient's life is to be saved. In other cases there is gradual narrowing of the intestine. As the narrowing increases the patient begins to complain of symptoms which get worse over a period of weeks or months. This condition is called subacute or chronic intestinal obstruction and although surgical treatment will be required there is no great urgency. Some patients with subacute intestinal obstruction suddenly develop acute intestinal obstruction and require immediate surgical relief.

Types of Intestinal Obstruction

1   *Paralytic Ileus*

The small intestine may be paralysed following the trauma of an abdominal operation and this tends to be marked and prolonged if there has been a lot of handling of the intestine. It is also paralysed following peritonitis and this is probably due to the toxic effects of the bacteria causing the peritonitis. The practical effect of paralytic ileus is that the patient has the clinical appearance of an obstruction because the paralysed intestine does not have any peristalsis.

2   *Mechanical Obstruction*

The small intestine is about 6 metres long and it may be obstructed anywhere along its length. Mechanical obstructions may be simple or complicated by strangulation. It is usual to divide the causes of mechanical obstruction into those within the lumen, those in the wall, and those compressing the intestine from outside.

(a)   Causes within the Lumen.   Simple mechanical obstruction can be caused by a large gallstone which has passed into the duodenum and down the intestine. This condition is called gallstone ileus and the stone usually stops and occludes the intestine about two feet above the caecum. Another cause is a food bolus. The patient is elderly and edentulous and often gives a history of eating an orange. Such a patient, unable to chew effectively, swallows at least half an orange in a single piece. The orange passes unaltered and blocks the lower ileum which is too small for it to pass any further. Intussusception is a condition is which the intestine telescopes into itself. It used to be common in infants but has now become rare and is sometimes seen as a complication of a small intestine tumour. Intussusception is a strangulated obstruction.

(b)   Causes in the Wall of the Intestine.   Regional ileitis or Crohn's disease causes subacute intestinal obstruction as the intestine narrows with the progress of the disease. Subacute obstruction is also caused by tumours arising in the wall of the intestine. Lymphoma and less commonly adenocarcinoma are tumours which may be responsible for subacute obstruction.

(c) Compression of the Intestine from Outside. A common cause of external compression is adhesions. These often follow a previous operation. Adhesions may also result from leaks of intestinal contents or from previous inflammation such as acute diverticulitis of the colon. Starch powder, which is used to lubricate surgical gloves, can cause adhesions and surgeons wash their gloved hands to remove starch powder before beginning an operation.

Inguinal and femoral hernia cause acute intestinal obstruction when the loop of intestine is compressed at the neck of the hernial sac. This is a strangulated type of obstruction because the blood vessels to the loop of intestine within the hernial sac are also compressed.

Volvulus or twisting of the intestine is more common in the large intestine. When it occurs the loop is occluded at its base. The blood vessels are also blocked by the twisting so that volvulus is a strangulated obstruction.

3   *Vascular Obstruction*

When there is a sudden occlusion of the main mesenteric artery by thrombosis or embolism the intestine becomes ischaemic and ceases to function. The clinical presentation is of acute strangulated intestinal obstruction.

Diagnosis of Intestinal Obstruction

There may be signs of dehydration such as a dry tongue, inelastic skin and hypotension. The abdominal symptoms and signs are very characteristic.

Colicky pain is a constant feature of intestinal obstruction. It is caused by the excessive peristalsis which results from attempts to overcome the obstruction and is accompanied by increased peristaltic sounds which may be audible.

Vomiting is usually an early feature of intestinal obstruction. It may be delayed when the obstruction is in the distal bowel and is early in high obstruction. Faeculent vomiting is usually a late sign. This brown, offensive smelling vomit is small intestinal fluid heavily infected with bacteria and containing altered blood. It is not faeces.

The patient may pass faeces which are located distal to the point of obstruction but when the obstruction is complete he will not pass faeces or flatus again until the obstruction is relieved.

As the intestines distend there will be corresponding distension of the abdomen.

In high obstruction there is excessive vomiting but very little intestinal and abdominal distension but when the obstruction is in the distal ileum there is massive distension but vomiting may be late.

Tenderness of the abdomen usually indicates an area of strangulation. Patients with a strangulated obstruction may pass blood from the rectum.

Radiography

Many cases of intestinal obstruction are so clinically obvious that radiography is not essential. However, most cases are X-rayed with the patient in the erect and supine positions. The erect films may be expected to show fluid levels in the distended bowel. If the patient is not well enough to stand, lateral films may be taken with the patient in a lateral position.

Physiological Changes in Acute Intestinal Obstruction

In simple mechanical obstruction the intestine above the point of obstruction becomes distended with air and fluid. The air comes from swallowed air which normally passes through the intestine and the fluid is a combination of bile, pancreatic and small intestinal secretions. This can amount to 10 litres a day so that there is a rapid accumulation of air and fluid. The normal absorption of fluid is reduced when the intestine is distended by obstruction and as a result the body loses fluid and also electrolytes such as sodium and potassium. This loss causes a clinical condition in the patient which is called dehydration. The tongue is dry, the eyes sunken and the skin loses its elasticity. The fluid lost into the intestine comes from the circulating blood. The fluid between the cells of the body (extracellular fluid) is drawn on to preserve the circulating blood volume and it is this loss of extracellular fluid which causes the signs of dehydration. As the condition worsens there is insufficient extracellular fluid to maintain the correct volume of fluid in the blood circulation and as the blood volume falls the patient begins to show signs of hypovolaemic shock (see Chapter 7).

When obstruction is complicated by strangulation the effects are more dramatic as there is an additional loss of blood and plasma into the strangulated intestine which increases the shock due to loss of the circulating blood volume.

Strangulation may also be complicated by septicaemic shock resulting from the absorption of bacterial toxins from the dead and infected intestine (see Chapter 7).

When a patient shows moderately severe signs of dehydration he has lost about 2–3 litres of normal saline from the body.

Management of Acute Intestinal Obstruction

Whatever the cause of acute intestinal obstruction treatment is first directed towards correction of the disturbance of fluid and electrolytes in the body.

Nasogastric Tube

This is usually passed in the ward and the stomach completely emptied. It is essential to empty the stomach before the patient goes to theatre because of the risk of vomiting and inhalation of gastric contents during induction of anaesthesia. Once the tube is in the stomach, gastric and upper intestinal distension is relieved and the patient ceases to vomit.

Intravenous Treatment

If a patient shows moderate clinical signs of dehydration he has lost at least 2 litres of normal saline. The patient will be given intravenous normal saline and the fluid may be given quickly so that the physiological state can be rapidly restored so making the subsequent operation safer. However, it is necessary to make a number of regular measurements to gather data on which the further prescription of fluids and electrolytes can be based.

1 A catheter is placed in the superior vena cava. This is called a central venous line and is used to measure the pressure in the region of the right atrium of the heart. This is a good indicator of the fluid requirement and fluid may be given rapidly until the central venous pressure (CVP) reaches its normal value of 10–12 cm of water. If too much fluid is given and the circulation overloaded the central venous pressure will be seen to rise before there is serious strain on the heart.

It is better to set up a separate intravenous infusion for the administration of fluid as there is a risk of infecting the CVP line if it is used for infusion. Although most of the fluid will consist of water and electrolytes, many patients with hypovolaemic shock require at least one unit of blood or plasma.

2   A urinary catheter is passed and connected to a collecting bag. In this way the output can be measured at regular intervals and should reach 60 ml in one hour, although in the acute phase the doctor will be satisfied with any output over 700 ml in 24 hours.

3   An immediate measurement of the blood urea and electrolytes is requested from the laboratory and this is repeated daily until the fluid and electrolyte situation is stable.

4   The intake and output are carefully measured and recorded on a fluid balance chart which is totalled and studied by the doctor every 12 or 24 hours so that an assessment of the requirements for the next 24 hours can be made.

Surgical Treatment

Once the patient's general condition is sufficiently improved, he is taken to the operating theatre for an operation to relieve the obstruction. The exact surgical procedure depends on the cause which is found at the operation.

A bolus obstruction or gallstone ileus is treated by opening the intestine where it is dilated just above the point of the obstruction and this is used to extract the cause of the obstruction. The incision is closed with catgut sutures. An intussusception is treated by reduction, but in some cases when the intussusception cannot be reduced it is necessary to do a resection and anastomosis.

Obstruction which is caused by a tumour growing in the wall of the intestine is usually treated by resecting the piece of intestine with the tumour and then anastomosing the ends of the intestine which remain. If the obstruction is caused by adhesions the surgeon divides the adhesions until the intestine is free and unobstructed. Inguinal and femoral herniae which are causing obstruction and strangulation are repaired after reduction or resection of the intestine in the hernial sac.

Postoperative Treatment of Intestinal Obstruction

Once an obstruction has been relieved by an operation it might be expected that the patient would have a smooth recovery. Unfortunately this is rarely the case because the distended intestine above the point of the obstruction is so stretched that it does not contract and the patient continues to have a functional obstruction.

Until such time as the intestine begins to contract he is maintained on intravenous fluid and electrolytes. The treatment at this stage is exactly as described in the section on management and the nurse has a great responsibility in the collection of data such as volume of urine output and gastric aspiration. The patient often wonders why he is not at once better and needs support and reassurance.

When the intestine recovers the doctor is able to hear peristaltic sounds with a stethoscope and the patient often notices gurgles from the abdomen. The passage of flatus from the rectum is a certain sign that recovery has taken place. At this point it is possible to introduce oral fluid and to remove the the gastric tube. It is wise to begin the oral fluid slowly on about 30 ml hourly and this may be increased rapidly. At the same time intravenous treatment becomes unnecessary.

It is best to nurse the patient with considerable periods sitting in a chair even in the early stages when he is on gastric drainage and intravenous fluid.

17

Appendicitis

The appendix is a narrow tubular part of the intestinal tract which is attached to the caecum. Although the point of attachment is constant the appendix may lie in any direction and the position of the appendix determines some of the presenting symptoms.

In appendicitis the appendix wall is infected with the mixed bacteria which normally live in the colon. The inflammatory response is the same as elsewhere in the body, causing swelling of the appendix. A few cases of appendicitis resolve but the majority continue until pus is formed. The pus is discharged into the lumen of the appendix and if it is obstructed by a small dehydrated fragment of faeces (a faecolith) the pus cannot escape along the lumen to drain into the caecum. This results in early perforation of the appendix and discharge of pus into the peritoneal cavity. This is what is meant by a ruptured or burst appendix and of course the spread of infection outside the lumen of the appendix makes the illness much more serious (Fig. 45). Hanging from a broad attachment to the transverse colon is an organ called the great omentum. This important organ has been variously named the 'fatty apron', because of its shape like an apron inside the abdomen, and the 'abdominal policeman' because of its function in moving towards and enveloping any infective process in the abdomen. If the great omentum successfully surrounds the appendix before it ruptures the infection will be localised to the area of the perforation. This will result in an appendix abscess, generally in the right iliac fossa. If the great omentum does not succeed in localising the infection the whole peritoneal cavity may be infected when the appendix perforates. This will result in the much more serious condition of peritonitis.

Treatment of Appendicitis

1   The most important part of the treatment of appendicitis is to remove the appendix (appendicectomy). This is usually done through what is called a gridiron incision in the right iliac fossa of the abdomen (Fig. 45). The wound will be drained if an abscess is present. In an early case this may be all the treatment that is necessary but other non-surgical measures are needed in some cases.

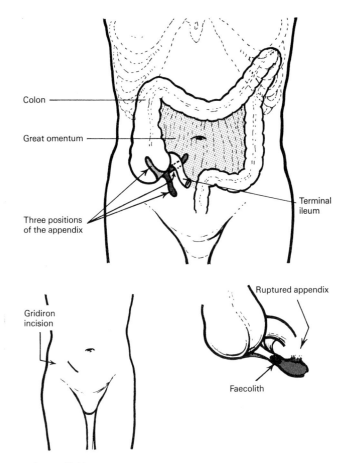

Colon

Great omentum

Three positions
of the appendix

Terminal
ileum

Gridiron
incision

Ruptured appendix

Faecolith

Fig 45 Appendicitis

2 *Antibacterial agents.* A number of different bacteria are involved in the infection and it is necessary to use two antibacterial agents to overcome them. Metronidazole is used to control the bacteroides and some other bacteria. This is best given by suppository as it is very effective by this route and well absorbed. In addition, it is usual at present to give a bacteriocidal drug in the cephalosporin group. Most of these need to be given by intravenous or intramuscular route but cephradine can be given by mouth.

The timing of antibacterial treatment is important as it is better to do the operation when there is a high level of drugs in the blood. To achieve this the drugs are given with the premedication and a further suppository of metronidazole may be given at the end of the operation.

3   If the patient has peritonitis it will be necessary to give fluid intravenously and to keep the stomach empty with a gastric tube. When the paralytic ileus recovers the surgeon will be able to hear normal intestinal sounds and the patient will pass wind rectally. At this time oral fluid can be started and the intravenous infusion taken down. Patients on intravenous therapy will have the cephalosporin intravenously through a burette but the metronidazole can still be given by suppository.

Complications

The most common complication of appendicitis is an abscess. This may occur in the abdominal wound, which becomes red and tender and eventually discharges pus. If the wound is tense the discharge may be encouraged by separating the wound edges and gently opening the abscess with forceps.

A more troublesome site of an abscess is inside the abdomen at the site of the appendix. The general signs of infection such as raised temperature and pulse rate are present. There may also be pain and tenderness in the right lower abdomen and after some days a lump can be felt. Discharge of pus through the wound is to be expected, but if the patient continues to be unwell and the abscess shows no sign of discharging it may be opened under an anaesthetic in the operating theatre.

Sometimes the infection gravitates down into the pelvis causing a pelvic abscess. This irritates the bladder and rectum causing frequency of micturition and diarrhoea. The pelvic abscess can be felt by the surgeon on rectal examination. Incision and drainage of a pelvic abscess is not often done because it usually discharges spontaneously through the rectum. The patient complains of diarrhoea and if the stool is kept for examination it may be seen to contain blood and mucus. When the abscess discharges into the rectum the patient will pass a stool which he describes as being very offensive and liquid. Once this has happened the patient's general condition improves dramatically. The abscess cavity is draining from its lowest point and clears up very quickly.

18

The Colon

Anatomy and Physiology

The colon, sometimes called the large intestine because it is wider in diameter than the small intestine, extends from the end of the small intestine to the anus. It is about 1½ metres in length. The colon runs round the periphery of the abdomen with the coils of small intestine in the centre. It begins in the lower right abdomen where the appendix is attached to it. The individual parts of the colon are shown in Figure 46.

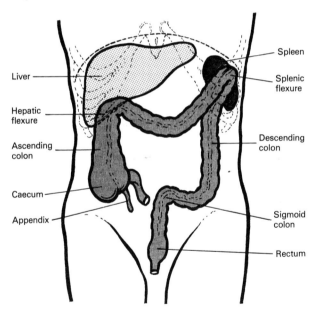

Fig 46   Anatomy of colon and rectum

The muscle layers are circular and longitudinal. The longitudinal muscle, which is on the outside, is arranged in bands called taenia. This muscle is shorter than the intestine which is puckered into saccules giving the colon a very characteristic appearance. Like all intestine the colon is lined with a cellular layer called the epithelium or mucosa. In the colon there are many tubular glands which are lined with cells including a large number which secrete mucus, which has the important function of lubricating the faeces. Muscular contractions convey the faeces gradually towards the distal colon but the muscle of the colon tends to contract massively at the time of defaecation so that the whole colon from the hepatic flexure empties.

The second important function of the colon is absorption of water so that the liquid content of the caecum becomes solid by the time it reaches the sigmoid colon. This conserves water in the body and people with diarrhoea become dehydrated.

Inflammatory Bowel Disease

Most of the diseases of the colon and rectum are inflammatory or neoplastic. There are two inflammatory diseases which are called ulcerative colitis and Crohn's disease of the colon. There is very little difference between these diseases as they present to the surgeon but they are in fact separate entities and have slightly different courses and prognosis.

Acute Ulcerative Colitis

Ulcerative colitis may present as an acute fulminating disease with up to 30 or more bowel actions daily. There is usually faecal incontinence and the faeces contain much blood and pus. Patients with this form of the disease lose so much fluid and electrolytes that they rapidly become dehydrated because of the passage of water from the extracellular fluid to make up the blood volume. Later, as the extracellular reserves of fluid are depleted, the blood volume cannot be kept up and the patient shows the signs of hypovolaemic shock. The colon is extensively ulcerated and may dilate and even perforate, causing faecal peritonitis which is usually fatal.

Chronic Ulcerative Colitis

The acute form may gradually turn into chronic colitis or the disease may present in this way. The patient has diarrhoea with blood and pus in the stools but the disease is much less severe than the acute form. There is a gradual loss of fluid and electrolytes and the loss of nutrition caused by the diarrhoea gradually induces a condition of cachexia.

The disease may affect a part of the colon or the whole colon when it is called total colitis. The complications of chronic colitis are:

1 Perianal complications such as abscess and fistula.

2 Carcinoma of the colon. This is a serious complication and occurs in about 10% of cases of total colitis which has been present more than 10 years.

3 The general cachectic state includes chronic dehydration, hypoproteinaemia, hypokalaemia and iron deficiency anaemia.

Investigations

Chronic cases are studied with barium enema and colonoscopy, but these investigations are dangerous during an acute attack.

Treatment

Acute Ulcerative Colitis. Early surgery carries a high mortality in the acute form of colitis and medical treatment is always given in the first place. Treatment takes several forms:

1 As the patient is suffering from hypovolaemic shock the first priority is to replace the fluid (including blood) by intravenous infusion.

2 Some form of antidiarrhoeal agent should be given such as codeine phosphate or Lomotil.

3 *Steroids* Systemic steroids are used in the acute phase and surgical treatment can usually be avoided.

4 *Surgical treatment* Surgery is reserved for patients who fail to show improvement with steroid therapy. Patients on steroid therapy may perforate the colon without any symptoms of perforation or peritonitis and if there is any doubt an X-ray of the abdomen should be taken. Perforation will be confirmed by the presence of gas in the abdomen. If surgical treatment is decided on it will consist of colectomy and ileostomy. If the patient is well enough the rectum is also removed but it may be left for later excision.

Chronic Ulcerative Colitis. Many patients are treated medically for years with general support and steroids in small doses. Salazopyrine is often used and there is evidence that it gives some control of the disease over a long period.

The indications for surgery are:

1 General nutritional state and cachexia so interferes with the

quality of life that it is decided that life with an ileostomy would be preferable.

2   In cases of more than 10 years duration and involving the whole colon the risk of carcinoma has to be taken into account. In this sort of case the surgeon is justified in putting more pressure on the patient to have a colectomy and ileostomy and the risks must be fully explained to the patient.

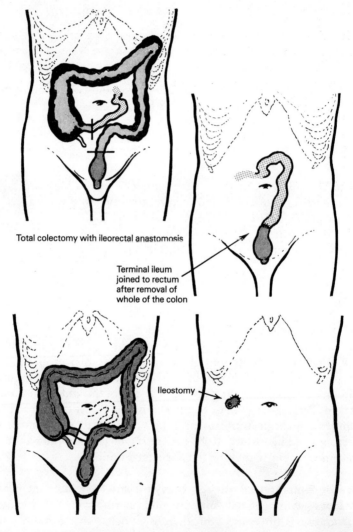

Total colectomy with ileorectal anastomosis

Terminal ileum joined to rectum after removal of whole of the colon

Ileostomy

Total proctocolectomy with ileostomy

Fig 47   Operations for inflammatory disease of colon

Surgical treatment may be proctocolectomy and permanent ileostomy or in some cases total colectomy with ileorectal anastomosis. Surgical opinion is divided about the correct choice of operation (Fig. 47).

Crohn's Disease of the Colon

Clinical Features. The clinical picture closely resembles that seen in chronic ulcerative colitis but acute fulminating disease is not seen in Crohn's colitis. The patient with Crohn's disease of the colon has diarrhoea with blood, mucus and pus in the stool and may gradually become cachectic.

Treatment. Many cases can be kept in reasonable health with conservative treatment and general supportive measures together with steroids and salazopyrine.

Surgical treatment is indicated when the degree of general ill health becomes intolerable and the surgeon and patient feel that life would be more tolerable after an operation. There is probably no risk of malignancy complicating Crohn's disease. This fact and the fact that the disease is often segmental means that the surgical approach can be more conservative than in ulcerative colitis and the rectum can often be preserved. The operations which can be done for Crohn's disease are:

1   right hemicolectomy for right colon disease with or without disease in the terminal ileum (Fig. 48);

2   total proctocolectomy and ileostomy for the rare case involving the whole colon;

3   colectomy with ileorectal anastomosis.

Preoperative Treatment of Colectomy for Inflammatory Disease

Usually the patient who is to be treated surgically is in poor general condition following many months or years of illness. The patient will generally require an intravenous infusion to restore the fluids and electrolytes. If he is anaemic, blood is transfused to bring the haemoglobin up to around 11 or 12 g and in some cases a short period of intravenous feeding will be required.

It is not possible to empty the bowel of a patient with severe and chronic diarrhoea but antibiotics will be needed before, during and

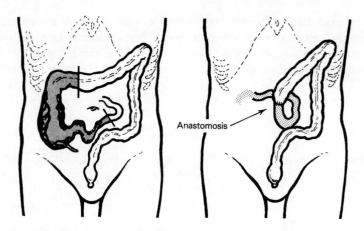

Fig 48   Ileocolectomy for right-sided inflammatory bowel disease

after the operation. These consist of a broad spectrum antibiotic and also metronidazole which is specific in the control of the colon bacteria called bacteroides.

Ileostomy

Ileostomy is the creation of an opening or stoma in the terminal ileum which is brought to the surface in the right lower abdomen. The problem is a significant one as it is estimated that there are about 15 000 people in England and Wales with an ileostomy. An ileostomy discharges ileal contents continuously throughout the day. As the ileal contents are fluid and contain digestive enzymes, there are particular problems about preventing the fluid which comes from an ileostomy from coming into contact with and digesting the skin. Skin which has been partly digested by ileal contents becomes red and painful, and discharges serum making the adhesion of any appliance more difficult.

All patients who have major and mutilating surgery suffer from some feeling of inadequacy in general and in sexual performance. When an ileostomy is added to this there is the additional dread of becoming a social outcast. The patient feels a repugnance at the thought of the discharge of faeces onto the abdominal wall and fears that he will be shunned by people because of constant smell. In younger patients there is also fear of repelling the opposite sex and of difficulty with sexual intercourse, pregnancy and childbearing. All of these fears are without foundation but it needs the support of all the hospital staff to give the patient confidence that with modern care and appliances he or she will be able to lead a virtually normal life.

An ileostomy is made as a spout of intestine about $1\frac{1}{2}$ inches long which projects from the abdominal wall into a bag which is stuck to the skin around the stoma. In this way the contents are directed into the bag without contact with the skin (Fig. 47). The actual detail of fixing a bag so that it will not leak has been a difficult problem. Many advances were made by members of the Ileostomy Association, which is a group of people with ileostomies who meet together to discuss their problems. In recent years great help for ileostomists has come from stoma therapists. In this country the stoma therapist is a nurse who has had additional training in the care and management of all types of stoma and whose work is entirely with patients with stomas.

Before the operation, the stoma therapist sees the patient and explains the operation and the subsequent management, doing everything possible to allay the patient's natural fears. Although the final decision concerning the exact siting of the ileostomy rests with the surgeon, the stoma therapist usually marks the proposed position on the abdominal wall. Bearing in mind that the bag has to stick to the skin, the stoma is sited away from a boney prominence and it must also avoid a skin crease which might result in a leak. The patient is sat up to ensure that in this position a crease does not appear at the site for the ileostomy. The ileostomy must be at least as high as the umbilicus as the bag hangs down and will cross the groin and kink when the patient sits if it is placed too low.

In the days of preparation before the operation the ward nurse has a vital role in supporting and encouraging the patient.

Postoperative Management of an Ileostomy

The great aim is to prevent leakage. If it occurs the patient will lose confidence in the system and also in the advisors who have been giving assurance that he will lead a normal life. In addition, once ileal contents come into contact with the skin it becomes inflamed and discharges fluid, making adhesion of the bag more difficult.

Two materials have contributed to the increased security of ileostomy bags. One is Stomahesive (Squibb) which is supplied in the form of a thin sheet which can be cut to the size required. Stomahesive is made from gelatin, pectin and a complicated form of cellulose. It is soft and can be moulded to the skin round the stoma and it will adhere even to moist inflamed skin.

The second material is karaya gum (Abbott Laboratories) which is a sticky brown material obtained from plants. Its most common use is in the form of a seal or washer incorporated in most ileostomy bags used at the present time. The karaya makes a firm adhesion and will stick to inflamed skin.

Theatre Management

At the conclusion of the operation, the diameter of the base of the stoma is measured and a karaya seal stoma bag of the correct size is fitted. The seal should be a snug fit so that there is no risk of leak or of pressure necrosis. The bag is fitted horizontally so that it hangs to the right side when the patient is lying in bed. Later when the patient is mobile the bag is fitted vertically.

Ward Management

The aim of ward management is to teach the patient to manage his own ileostomy before going home. Blind patients and those with severe arthritis may not be able to manage on their own and in these cases the services of a close relative has to be sought.

Although the stoma therapist will give frequent advice, the actual care falls to the ward nurse who is responsible for the total care of the patient. The bag should be emptied when about half full. The patient should not need to ask for the bag to be emptied as he may find this embarrassing and the nurse must see that the bag never overfills.

Types of Bag

There have been many improvements in recent years and a number of appliances in use only a few years ago are now obsolete. The appliances in current use may be in one or two pieces. The one piece bag consists of a karaya gum washer to which the bag is attached. The bag may be closed or open at the bottom (Fig. 56). The open type is closed with a plastic clip. The closed bag has to be completely changed each time it is filled and is quite unsuitable for an ileostomy. The one piece bag which is closed with a clip may be emptied into a bowl if the patient is still in bed or into the toilet if he is ambulant.

The bag is then washed and the clip replaced. The two piece bag consists of a karaya seal with a flange which is left attached to the skin for up to a week. The bags have an elasticated opening which fits over the flange making it easy to change the bag when necessary.

In changing the bag, the nurse must try to get the patient to look at and to accept this unusual new piece of anatomy as soon as possible. The longer this is put off the more difficult it becomes. When the bag is removed from the skin the area is washed with soap and water and dried with a tissue. Slight bleeding from a stoma is not unusual and should not be cause for concern. The ileum often looks a little blue for a few days but this need not cause any anxiety.

If there is a small area of leakage under the bag it is tempting to try to patch this in some way. This is absolutely contraindicated as ileal contents are in contact with, and damaging, the skin. If there is any sign of leakage the bag must be changed.

One of the more difficult problem is the distension of the bag with flatus. Some bags have an incorporated disc which releases gas and absorbs the faecal smell, but this solution is not really satisfactory and further study is needed. Other patients prefer to make a pinhole in the bag and to cover it with a piece of Elastoplast which they lift to let out wind at a convenient moment.

If soreness develops around an ileostomy it can often be cured by applying a sheet of Stomahesive snugly round the stoma and attaching the karaya seal to the Stomahesive.

By the time the patient is discharged he must be able to take full care of his ileostomy.

Home Care of an Ileostomy

Although the patient comes under the care of the general practitioner when he is at home, he usually retains the telephone number of the stoma therapist whom he is able to consult. Stoma therapists make home visits if necessary. The patient will take home sufficient bags and materials to keep him going for some time and after that the general practitioner will prescribe for him. All bags and other materials needed for the care of stomas are provided free of charge by the National Health Service.

In general discussion the patient should be told that he may expect to lead a virtually normal life. There need be no change in normal sexual intercourse, and pregnancy and normal delivery is quite usual in younger women.

There need not be any dietary restrictions, but if the patient finds that the ileostomy is upset by a particular article of food it is obviously wise to avoid this in future. Fluid loss from an ileostomy amounts to about 750 ml daily and patients should be encouraged to drink well to make up this deficit.

Although the ileostomy bags are supposed to be disposable, the patients need advice about this. They are told not to dispose of bags in the toilet as this often results in blocking the drain. The bags are wrapped in newspaper and placed in a refuse bag or bin.

Patients with an ileostomy usually wear their bag while taking a bath, as there is a possibility that the ileostomy may discharge into the water. For women it is possible to disguise an appliance with a onepiece bathing costume and men are advised to wear shorts over their swimming trunks.

Continent Ileostomy

This new development of ileostomy is still in the experimental stage. At the operation a reservoir with a valve is constructed from several loops of terminal ileum. The patient is taught to empty the intestine by passing a tube at certain fixed intervals. Such a patient docs not need to wear a bag but at the present time the technique is still being studied and developed.

Diverticulitis

A diverticulum is a small pouch attached to the colon. Usually diverticula are multiple. Though most common in the sigmoid colon they may involve the whole of the large intestine.

The term diverticulosis implies the presence of multiple diverticula without complications and often diagnosed as an incidental finding on X-ray. Diverticulitis means that the diverticula are infected. The term 'diverticular disease' is often used in X-ray reports. It means that the radiologist has found diverticula to be present but on the evidence of the X-ray it is not possible to say if infection is present or not.

Diverticulosis is an aquired abnormality. It is more common in men and occurs in obese patients in middle age. Although diverticulosis may be very extensive diverticulitis is rarely seen except in the sigmoid colon.

Diverticula occur in rows emerging from the colon at the same point as shown in Fig. 49. The neck of the diverticulum is closely related to the artery supplying the colon and this accounts for the

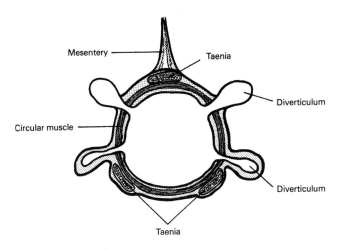

Fig 49 Diverticula of colon

occasional complication of severe haemorrhage. The colon is often contracted with a strong, thick muscle coat and a narrow lumen, a fact which is often attributed to the low roughage diet of Europeans.

Diverticulosis is very common and does not cause any serious symptoms. However, the diverticula often contain a hard, dehydrated fragment of faeces called a faecolith and infection with faecal bacteria may begin in such a diverticulum. Infection often occurs in a group of diverticula at the same time giving rise to the clinical condition of acute diverticulitis. The patient complains of constant severe pain in the left iliac fossa and the abdomen is tender on palpation. The condition resembles left-sided appendicitis and is usually easy to diagnose. In more severe infections, perforation of at least one diverticulum takes place liberating faecal bacteria into the surrounding tissues. Often this infection is confined, giving rise to an abscess alongside the colon which is called a paracolic abscess. In more dramatic cases the perforation is into the general peritoneal cavity which is flooded with faecal pus and in the worst cases with faeces. This is called perforated diverticulitis with peritonitis. Perforation of the colon is characterised by the presence of a large amount of gas in the peritoneum and this may be seen on an X-ray film. More important is the fact that the patient will rapidly become seriously ill. Bacteria are absorbed from the peritoneal cavity into the blood stream causing what is called Gram-negative septicaemia, because the bacteria give a Gram-negative stain when examined in the laboratory. Another term which is used is 'septicaemic shock', which is the clinical condition resulting from this type of septicaemia and which is described in Chapter 7.

Treatment of Acute Diverticulitis

Many cases of diverticulitis are treated conservatively in hospital or even at home. The main treatment is the use of the antibacterial agent metronidazole (Flagyl) which is particularly lethal to colon bacteria. During the acute phase the patient will be treated with fluids.

If a paracolic abscess or perforated diverticulitis is diagnosed surgery will be necessary.

Preoperative Management

The patient is certain to have peritonitis and will have inactive intestines (paralytic ileus) until the peritonitis is cured. He will therefore be unable to take oral fluid and an intravenous infusion is begun. The exact fluid infused will depend on the degree of dehydration and the results of an emergency estimation of the blood electrolytes. The doctors will have to warn the patient of the probability of a colostomy and if he is too ill the relatives must be informed.

An intravenous broad spectrum antibiotic is used. Metronidazole can also be given intravenously but is expensive and it is safe and effective to give it by suppository either into the rectum or after the operation into the rectum or colostomy.

Operative Management

During the operation the anaesthetist will pass a nasogastric tube. The surgery is illustrated in Fig. 50. A proximal transverse colostomy and a drain to the site of abscess or perforation is the easiest and quickest operation. However, the faeces between the site of the colostomy and the leak at the site of perforation continue to discharge through the perforation and there is a very high mortality from this operation. Many surgeons try to prevent this by resecting the acutely inflamed and perforated intestine and establishing an end colostomy which can be closed at a later operation.

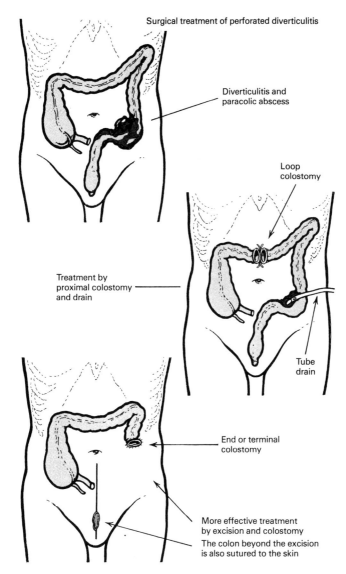

Surgical treatment of perforated diverticulitis

Diverticulitis and
paracolic abscess

Loop
colostomy

Treatment by
proximal colostomy
and drain

Tube
drain

End or terminal
colostomy

More effective treatment
by excision and colostomy
The colon beyond the excision
is also sutured to the skin

Fig 50   Surgical treatment of perforated diverticulitis

Postoperative Management

The patient has peritonitis and ileus and the treatment consists of
antibacterial agents including metronidazole and strict attention to
the fluid balance. The colostomy is covered with a drainable bag, but

there will be no action until intestinal function recovers. Passage of wind from the colostomy will be the first sign and this will inflate the bag. Once intestinal function returns the nasogastric tube can be removed and oral fluids can be introduced as intravenous fluid is phased out.

As with all colostomy patients, there is need for much support and encouragement, though with such a serious illness the patient usually accepts the colostomy as the price of life. Provided the surgeon is optimistic about closure he can be encouraged to believe that the colostomy will be closed in about 2−3 months.

Haemorrhage

Sometimes a patient with diverticulitis will present with acute rectal bleeding, which is often sufficient to need treatment with blood transfusion. The bleeding is caused by damage to a small artery which runs close to the neck of a diverticulum. The bleeding usually stops and surgical intervention is not generally required.

Vesicocolic Fistula

This is an opening between the colon and the bladder. It is sometimes caused by a cancer of the colon which has invaded the bladder, but diverticulitis is by far the most common cause. An abscess forms between the colon and the bladder. It is already in communication with the colon from which it has arisen and a fistula occurs if the abscess ruptures into the bladder. Strangely there is often no clear history of an acute attack of diverticulitis but the abscess arises quietly and the diagnosis is only made when it ruptures into the bladder. It is unusual for urine to run into the rectum and be passed with the stools. Generally the hole is small and gas passes from the colon to the bladder giving rise to the symptom of passage of air in the urine, which is called pneumaturia. Of course the bladder is infected with colon bacteria, but symptoms of cystitis are rarely prominent and the main or only symptom is pneumaturia.

Vesicocolic fistula is treated by an operation in which the bladder is separated from the colon and the hole in each is repaired. The pre and postoperative management does not differ from that of all colonic surgery but a catheter is left in the bladder for about 10 days. During this time the bladder remains empty and the usual filling and emptying does not take place. With the bladder immobilised the sutured opening in it has a chance to heal.

Chronic Diverticulitis

Many patients come to the doctor with recurrent pain in the left lower abdomen. This situation is very different from the acute and dangerous one which exists in acute diverticulitis. The patient is not ill but complains of pain and the main concern of the doctor is to exclude a cancer of the colon which may present with similar pain in the same part of the abdomen. It is perfectly safe and indeed necessary to investigate such a case by doing a barium enema and colonoscopy. The barium enema shows a very characteristic picture as the barium fills the diverticula alongside the colon.

Tumours of the Colon and Rectum

Some colorectal tumours are benign but it is the malignant tumours which occupy so much of a surgeon's time.

Benign Tumours

1   **Juvenile Polyp.**   The juvenile polyp, which is seen in infants and children, is a malformation rather than a true tumour, though it appears as a tumour up to 1 cm in diameter on a stalk. Some of these disappear spontaneously but many are removed by ligation of the stalk because they bleed or prolapse through the anus on defaecation.

2   **Congenital polyposis** is a familial condition in which the baby is born with the inherited tendency to produce colorectal polyps. The polyps begin to appear at about the age of 12 to 14 years and by the age of 20 there may be hundreds of polyps throughout the colon and rectum. Unfortunately these polyps show a very marked tendency to convert to a malignant form and without treatment the patient will have multiple colon and rectal cancers by the age of 25 to 30. Early death is inevitable without treatment.

Children of families showing this disorder are observed by annual colonoscopy from the age of 13 or 14. If polyps appear the only course which is open to the surgeon is removal of the whole colon and rectum. This leaves the patient with a permanent ileostomy. Some surgeons advise leaving a short length of rectum to which the ileum can be anastomosed. This avoids an ileostomy life but the possibility of cancer developing in the rectal stump is very real and regular observation with diathermy destruction of polyps will be necessary.

3   The **adenomatous polyp** is a true tumour. It is benign at first but tumours which reach a diameter of 2 cm are often malignant and

eventual malignant change is common. These tumours cause rectal bleeding and are diagnosed by barium enema or colonoscopy. Treatment is essential because of the premalignant nature of the tumour. Small tumours can often be snared and removed using a colonoscope (Fig. 7). Larger tumours and those which may be malignant are approached by opening the abdomen. The tumour is felt through the colon and the bowel is opened to gain access and to remove the tumour. The colon is then closed with sutures.

4   The **villous papilloma** is different in structure but also presents with rectal bleeding. Passage of mucus is a marked feature. Mucus has a high content of potassium and the loss of so much mucus may result in a low blood potassium (hypokalaemia). The villous papilloma has a notorious reputation for being premalignant and early removal is essential. Diagnosis is by barium enema and colonoscopy when a biopsy diagnosis may be made.

Treatment

The technique for removal depends on the site and size of the tumour. Small and low tumours in the rectum may be removed through the anus. Larger tumours and those situated too high for removal through the anus are removed by a conservative resection of the rectum using the staple gun for a low anastomosis.

Tumours situated in the colon are usually treated by a resection of the piece of bowel from which the tumour is arising.

Malignant tumours of the Colon and Rectum

This is a relatively common type of cancer with an annual incidence of 20—30 new cases per 100 000 population. More than half of these cases are cancer of the rectum. The disease is most common in Europeans but rare in Africans and Asians. The highest incidence in the world is in north-east Scotland.

Cancer of the colon and rectum arises in the mucous membrane lining the intestine and is an adenocarcinoma. Many cases arise in previously existing benign adenoma or villous papilloma. About 10 % of patients with long standing total ulcerative colitis and patients with familial polyposis develop cancer of the colon and rectum but this accounts for a very small proportion of cases.

The behaviour, presentation and treatment varies according to the site of the cancer and it is usual to describe cancer of the right colon, of the left colon, and of the rectum.

Carcinoma of the Right Colon (Fig. 51)

The right colon is the caecum, ascending colon and hepatic flexure. This is a capacious part of the colon capable of stretching to a considerable diameter. Its contents are normally fluid and similar to

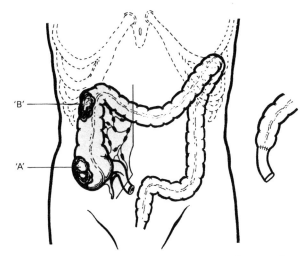

Carcinoma of the caecum 'A' or ascending colon 'B' are treated by right hemicolectomy. The nodes are removed with the intestine and after resection the ends are joined together with sutures

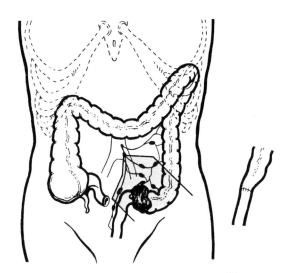

The operation which is done for carcinoma of the sigmoid colon. After resection the ends are sutured together

Fig 51 Operations for cancer of the colon

the content of the terminal ileum. Cancer in this part of the bowel tends to grow into the lumen as a large papillary tumour. Because of these features there is not usually any obstruction to the passage of the fluid content of the caecum past a tumour which does not encircle the bowel until a late stage. However, a large bulky tumour tends to bleed into the lumen and to cause the patient to become anaemic as a result of blood loss. The blood is usually so mixed with the faeces that it is not macroscopically obvious, although of course an occult blood test on the faeces will be positive. There are often no bowel symptoms and the patient goes to the doctor because of the symptoms which result from a chronic anaemia. These include pallor, shortness of breath on exertion, and a general feeling of malaise.

Cancer of the Transverse and Left Colon (Fig. 51)

This includes the colon from the hepatic flexure to the rectum. Two features determine the presentation of cancer of the left colon. One of the functions of the colon is absorption and conservation of water. This converts the liquid faeces of the right colon to solid faeces in the left side. Cancer of the left colon tends to grow round the circumference of the colon and this circumferential growth combined with the solid content makes it difficult for the faecal content to pass the cancer. As a result the patient complains of colicky abdominal pain as the colon above the growth contracts strongly to push the faeces past the obstruction. Eventually the faeces get stuck in the narrow stricture caused by the cancer and the patient presents to the doctor with acute intestinal obstruction. This is very similar to acute small intestine obstruction, which has already been described, but because the obstruction is so far down the intestinal tract there is a great deal of distended bowel above the obstruction and distension of the abdomen is marked feature.

Most patients with cancer of the left colon present with an altered bowel caused by the intermittent passage of faeces through the narrow segment of bowel. Passage of blood and mucus which is produced by the cancer is also a characteristic feature.

Cancer of the Rectum

When the cancer is growing in the rectum the patient notices blood and mucus streaking the stool. Another characteristic feature is a feeling of incomplete defaecation. This is caused by the growth in the rectum, which the patient interprets as faeces. Continued attempts to pass a stool when the rectum contains a carcinoma results in perineal pain and the passage of only blood and mucus. This symptom is called tenesmus.

Diagnosis of Colorectal Cancer

The diagnosis is often made on clinical examination and when the cancer is in the rectum it can be felt if the doctor does a rectal examination. If the cancer is in the rectum it can be seen and a biopsy taken with a proctoscope. Tumours out of range of the proctoscope may be reached and biopsied in the outpatient department with a steel sigmoidoscope which is 30 cm in length. Patients who are suspected of having a colonic cancer but who have a negative rectal examination and sigmoidoscopy are further investigated by barium enema. This usually gives a certain result but in some cases a colonoscopy may be done.

Spread of Colorectal Cancer

All forms of cancer spread in several ways. Direct invasion of adjacent structures often involves the posterior abdominal wall and it may also invade a loop of adjacent small intestine so that the colon with its cancer becomes attached by tumour to a piece of small intestine. Both of these forms of local invasion make operative removal more difficult but not impossible as the surgeon may be able to remove the main tumour with the attached structures in a single piece. The rectum is placed deep in the pelvis and local spread of cancer to the surrounding structures carries particular clinical problems both at the time of the initial presentation and in the event of local recurrence in the pelvis following surgical excision of the rectum. In front, the cancer may invade and become attached to the prostate and bladder in the male and to the posterior wall of the vagina in the female. In both sexes, involvement of the ureters may result in their obstruction causing uraemia because the urine cannot escape from the kidneys. Behind the rectum the sacrum and the nerves of the sacral plexus may be involved. Involvement of the nerves of the sacral plexus causes pain in the perineum and down the legs which is continuous and severe. The second way in which colon cancer spreads is through the lymph vessels to the local lymph nodes. The doctor can get some idea of the prognosis of a particular case by assessing how much it has advanced. This is called Dukes' staging after the pathologist who introduced it in cases of cancer of the rectum. It is now used in all cases of cancer of the colon and rectum. In stage A the tumour is confined to the wall of the bowel and in stage B it has spread to the structures outside. When the growth has spread to involve the lymph nodes the case is stage C (Fig. 52). In addition the cancer cells may enter the blood vessels in the tumour and be carried by the portal blood system to the liver where they are arrested in the capillary circulation of the liver. Such cells or groups of cells grow to form liver secondaries. Cancer cells may also be shed from the surface of the growth into the peritoneal cavity where they grow on the peritoneum to form little secondary nodules of growth. These nodules usually give rise to fluid which collects in the peritoneal cavity and this is called malignant ascites.

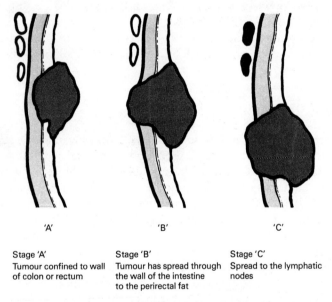

'A'   'B'   'C'

Stage 'A'
Tumour confined to wall of colon or rectum

Stage 'B'
Tumour has spread through the wall of the intestine to the perirectal fat

Stage 'C'
Spread to the lymphatic nodes

Fig 52 Dukes' pathological classification of colon and rectal cancer

Treatment of Cancer of the Colon

The only available treatment for cancer of the colon is surgical removal and the operation varies according to the site of the tumour. The operations are illustrated in Fig. 51. The principles are to remove the primary tumour together with the tissue alongside and also the mesentery containing the lymph nodes which drain lymph from the tumour and which may contain cancer cells. When there are liver secondaries the surgeon may still decide to resect the primary tumour even though prognosis is hopeless. This is called a palliative operation and is done to make the patient more comfortable and also to prevent the disaster of intestinal obstruction. In some cases the tumour is so fixed that it cannot be removed, or metastases in the liver and peritoneum are so extensive that it is not worthwhile.

Treatment of Cancer of the Rectum

Although some advanced cases have been treated by radiotherapy or chemotherapy it is generally considered that surgical treatment is the

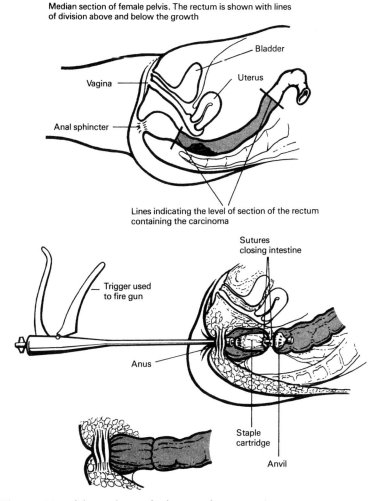

Fig 53   Use of the staple gun for low rectal anastomosis

only one which is effective. Removal of the whole rectum is called abdominoperineal resection of the rectum because part of the rectum is mobilised through an abdominal incision and the rest is approached through an incision which encircles the anus on the perineum. In such an operation an alternative opening for the faeces has to be made. This is called a colostomy and consists of attaching the end of the colon to the skin in the left side of the abdomen.

Colostomy is obviously distasteful to the patient and if the tumour is situated in the upper part of the rectum the whole operation can be performed through an abdominal incision. The lower part of the rectum and the anus are left and the colon brought down to and joined to the rectal stump. This is called a conservative resection. It can be done with sutures but is technically difficult and leakage is so common that a temporary colostomy is often made to divert the faeces until the sutured bowel is healed. The colostomy can be closed after a few weeks. Some tumours are so low in the rectum that it is impossible to suture the bowel together after excision. This problem is overcome by using a special instrument which inserts a row of steel staples to join the two pieces of intestine. This instrument is called a staple gun, because after putting it in position it is 'fired' by pressing a trigger (Fig. 53).

Intestinal Obstruction caused by Cancer of the Colon

The physiological changes which occur are the same as those seen in small bowel obstruction and the general measures needed to restore the body fluids to normal are the same and are fully described in Chapter 16. Once the patient is judged to be well enough an operation is undertaken to relieve the obstruction and sometimes to remove the tumour at the same time. The operations are illustrated in Fig. 54. A temporary or permanent colostomy is commonly made in the course of an operation for acute obstruction.

Preoperative Management of Cases of Colon and Rectal Cancer

As far as the patient is concerned the main anxiety is the possibility that he will return from the operation with a colostomy. In some cases the patient has to be told that a colostomy is inevitable and in others

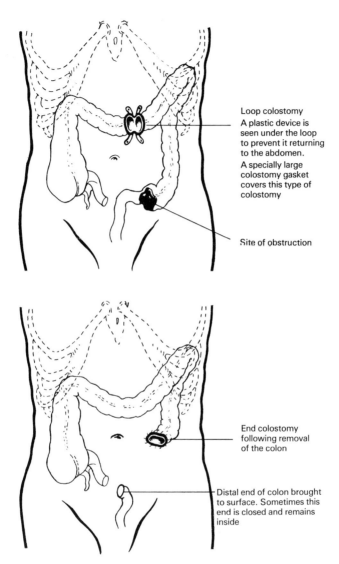

Loop colostomy
A plastic device is
seen under the loop
to prevent it returning
to the abdomen.
A specially large
colostomy gasket
covers this type of
colostomy

Site of obstruction

End colostomy
following removal
of the colon

Distal end of colon brought
to surface. Sometimes this
end is closed and remains
inside

Fig 54 Operations for large intestine obstruction

that it is a possibility, depending on the findings at the operation. The
patient may also be told that the colostomy will be permanent but in
some cases it will be possible to promise closure of the colostomy at a
later date. All patients dread a colostomy and often ask if they are
destined to wear a bag. Much of this fear stems from the days when
colostomy care was unsatisfactory. Modern colostomy management

is probably very different from what the patient believes and doctors and nurses have to do their best to persuade the patient that a colostomy life is very little different from normal. The two practical problems involved in large bowel surgery concern the presence of faeces in the bowel and the highly infective nature of the contents.

There are a number of techniques in use for clearing faeces from the intestine and it is essential that nurses and doctors fully discuss the preparation so that both know what is required. Some of the techniques are very unpleasant for the patient and the nurse should comment to the surgeon on problems which she experiences. The traditional technique for clearing the faeces is a combination of aperients and enemas. In recent years the traditional type of enema has been replaced by the small phosphate enema. In many centres the nurses may still be asked to employ this preparation but the bowel clearance is unreliable and often incomplete. For this reason surgeons have introduced other techniques. Obviously diet is important and two or even three days of fluid intake is often prescribed, though doctors may forget that this is quite a hardship for some patients. One technique in use is a total intestinal washout with normal saline. A gastric tube is passed and up to 10 litres of normal saline are introduced into the stomach over a period of some hours in the form of a drip feed. The patient is seated on a commode and as the saline passes through the intestine the patient's bowels open. At first this is normal but at the end of the procedure he should be passing clear normal saline. There are two objections to this mode of preparation. One is that it is a very trying procedure for the patient. The second is that some saline will be absorbed and this will cause an increase in the blood volume. Patients with cardiac failure or those with incipient failure may get serious cardiac symptoms as a result. Another way in which the colon can be cleared is with mannitol. This is given by mouth as 500 ml of 10% solution. It is not particularly unpalatable but can be flavoured with orange juice. Again the patient sits on a commode or has immediate access to one. The first bowel action takes place after about one hour and the washout is completed in about four hours. Mannitol is a substance which exerts a high osmotic pressure and water is drawn into the intestine as the mannitol passes through. This has the opposite effect to the saline washout because the patient is dehydrated. Using this preparation the patient should be given a high fluid intake before and after the preparation to combat the dehydrating effect of the mannitol. Another possible problem with mannitol is that it causes an excessive production of methane in the intestine. This is an explosive gas which might ignite if diathermy is used to open the intestine. Normal colon gas may also be explosive and it has been taught for many years that the colon should not be opened with diathermy because of this risk. An advantage is that mannitol preparation is not particularly trying for the patient.

The second consideration in the preoperative preparation is the control of infection by the bacteria normally present in the bowel. These are many and varied but most surgeons ask for some broad spectrum antibiotic. In addition it is essential to use metronidazole (Flagyl) as this is specific for anaerobic bacteria including one called bacteroides which is not sensitive to other antibiotics. The timing of the use of antibiotics is important as contamination takes place during the operation and may result in an active spreading infection so that the antibiotics and chemotherapy should be given with the premedication. Many surgeons also prescribe a second injection of antibiotic during the operation so that there is a high level in the blood at the time of the first contamination.

Postoperative Management of Operations on the Colon

The patient will return to the ward with an intravenous infusion and a gastric tube. These are managed in the usual way keeping the patient on intravenous fluids until there are signs of return of intestinal function. This is shown by the return of intestinal sounds which can be heard with a stethoscope and the passage of flatus. The patient is usually aware of gurgling sounds in the abdomen at this time. Once the patient's intestinal function has recovered oral fluids can be gradually introduced and the intravenous becomes unnecessary. Antibiotic cover is usually continued for five days.

Early mobility is usually recommended and there is no reason why the patient should not sit out on the day following the operation.

Most surgeons employ a drain following a colonic anastomosis. The drain is used as there is a small but real incidence of leakage from a colonic anastomosis. It usually occurs about the sixth or seventh day so that the drain is left in place for six or seven days but the surgeon's advice should always be sought. If there is any drainage it is likely to be smelly because of infection with anaerobic colonic bacteria. It is important to distinguish between faeculent pus and an actual faecal fistula or leak of faeces from the anastomosis along the tube. Most cases turn out to be faeculent pus but the matter can always be resolved by giving the patient a dye by mouth and if this does not appear colouring the discharge it is not a fistula. If a fistula does occur it usually closes and provided there is a track to the outside the patient's general condition will not deteriorate. However, if a leak occurs into the peritoneal cavity the patient will become ill and a temporary colostomy above the anastomosis will be required to allow the leak to heal without the problem of contamination with highly infected faeces.

Postoperative Management of Operations on the Rectum

The postoperative management is similar to that following colonic operations. The question of leakage is a more significant problem following conservative resections of the rectum when there has been a low anastomosis and awareness of this possibility is necessary. A protective colostomy is sometimes made following a difficult low rectal anastomosis. In these cases a barium examination of the rectum is done after about three weeks to make certain that there is no leak and if this is confirmed the colostomy can be closed.

Following resection of the rectum there is a possibility of temporary damage to the nerve supply of the bladder. This may cause difficulty with micturition so that a catheter is always placed in the bladder at the time of the operation. Some blood staining of the urine is common in the first 24 hours but it should always be reported. It usually results from minor bruising to the lining of the bladder caused by retraction during the operation rather than to any serious injury to the urinary tract. The catheter is removed on about the fifth morning after consultation with the medical staff.

In cases of abdominoperineal resection of the rectum in which the whole rectum and anus have been removed, the perineal wound is closed with sutures and one or two suction drains are left in the wound. These drains allow blood and fluid to pass without the need for frequent redressing of the wound. They are removed when drainage stops, usually about the fifth day.

Colostomy

A colostomy may be permanent or temporary. A temporary colostomy is usually made as a loop colostomy in which a loop is brought to the surface and retained in position by placing a plastic device under the intestine (Fig. 55). Some surgeons fear that faeces

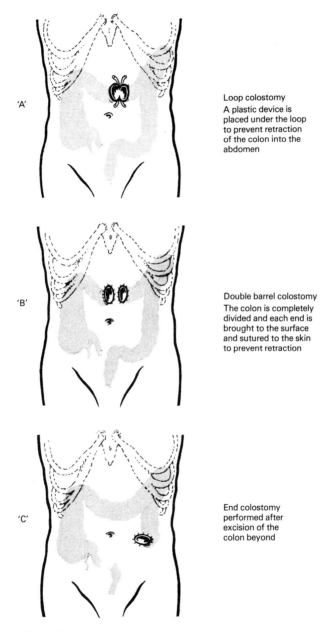

'A'

Loop colostomy
A plastic device is
placed under the loop
to prevent retraction
of the colon into the
abdomen

'B'

Double barrel colostomy
The colon is completely
divided and each end is
brought to the surface
and sutured to the skin
to prevent retraction

'C'

End colostomy
performed after
excision of the
colon beyond

Fig 55 Types of colostomy

may pass across this opening and therefore divide the intestine and bring the two ends out through two separate openings. This is called a double barrel colostomy. Its advantage in deviating the faeces is countered by the considerably greater difficulty in closure.

The permanent colostomy is usually in the sigmoid colon. The lining of the intestine is sutured to the skin to make a flush opening of the intestine.

Colostomy is a great problem and more than 100 000 people in Great Britain have a permanent colostomy requiring life-long management. The management of colostomy differs from that of ileostomy. The faeces tend to be liquid immediately after the operation but at least half the patients eventually return to one or two bowel actions a day so that the patient does not have to cope with constant filling of the colostomy bag with faeces. The second difference from ileostomy is that the contents of the colon are not markedly irritant or digestive so that there is no need for a spout.

In spite of all the recent advances in colostomy management and the appointment of stoma therapists patients still dread colostomy and need very strong support before and immediately following operation.

The siting of the colostomy is determined before the operation and marked on the skin. It is especially necessary in obese patients to study the proposed position with the patient sitting as well as lying down and as with ileostomy the stoma must not be near a boney prominence or skin crease which will cause diffficulties with bag attachment.

Management in the Operating Theatre

At the completion of the operation a drainable bag with a karaya gum washer is attached to the skin round the colostomy. The size should be an accurate fit. Too tight a fit may damage the bowel and a space between the colon and the washer will expose skin to the irritating effect of faeces. At this time the bag is fitted laterally as it lies more comfortably with the patient in bed.

Postoperative Ward Management

It is unusual for a colostomy to work for a few days. When it begins to work the faeces are liquid and the bag must not be allowed to get more than half-full. It is emptied into a receptacle by taking off the clip at the bottom. The liquid contents and need for frequent emptying at this stage is the reason that a drainable bag is used. The complete bag will need to be changed after four or five days. Before the patient leaves hospital he should be using a disposable bag which is non-drainable and he must be able to look after his own colostomy. When necessary the bag is changed. The contents are emptied into the toilet and the bag wrapped in newspaper and placed in the refuse bin. After washing and drying the skin a new bag is fitted (Fig. 56).

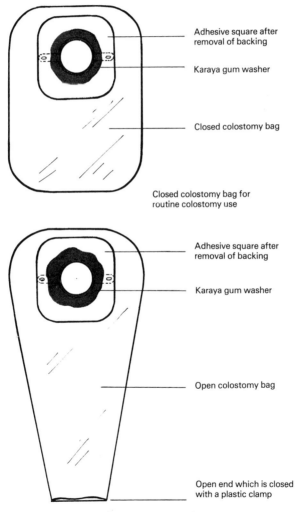

Adhesive square after removal of backing

Karaya gum washer

Closed colostomy bag

Closed colostomy bag for routine colostomy use

Adhesive square after removal of backing

Karaya gum washer

Open colostomy bag

Open end which is closed with a plastic clamp

Fig 56 Open colostomy bag for use immediately after the operation when the colostomy produces liquid faeces. This bag can also be used for an ileostomy

There are no special rules about diet, but if any article of food is found to cause diarrhoea it is best avoided. Some patients find that a daily dose of Isogel is helpful.

Colostomy Irrigation

Some patients never get regular colostomy actions and fear activity at inconvenient times. The irrigation technique has been reintroduced to try to help these patients. This method was recommended to patients 50 years ago but became unpopular because of complications. It is now popular in the USA but not in this country, possibly because of the cost of bags which are free in Great Britain. In the irrigation technique the patient uses a special apparatus with which he is able to fill the colon with water through the stoma. The water is returned with faeces over a period of up to one hour. Patients find that the technique takes altogether about 1½ hours but need be done only twice weekly. In between irrigations the patient wears a small pad to cover the stoma.

Late Problems

Most patients keep in touch with the stoma therapist for a time after discharge and later see her if there are any problems. It is necessary to tell patients that they can lead a virtually normal life as far as the colostomy is concerned. Fifty percent of men who have had a resection of the rectum are impotent. This is caused by damage to certain nerves in the pelvis and is not related to the colostomy which in itself does not interfere with sex or childbirth. Most operations for cancer are done on patients who are over 60.

As the colostomy is unlikely to work patients usually bath without a bag on the stoma.

19

The Anal Canal

Anatomy and Physiology (Fig. 57)

The anal canal is the last 3.5 cm of the intestine and is encircled by a ring of muscle called the anal sphincter which controls the exit of faeces from the rectum. The anal sphincter consists of two rings. The inner ring lies just under the surface and is called the internal sphincter. The external sphincter lies outside the internal sphincter. Part of the sphincter can be divided without interfering with continence but if the whole sphincter is divided the patient will be incontinent. Partial division may result in some degree of incontinence.

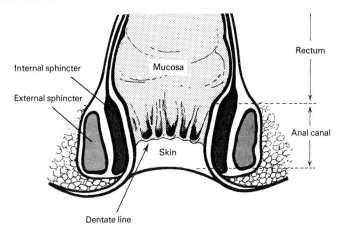

Fig 57 Anatomy of the anal canal and sphincters

The skin of the buttock extends into the anal canal for about half its length. Above this the lining is mucosa and is continuous with the mucosa of the rectum. The junction is easily seen with a proctoscope as an irregular line which is called the dentate line. This line has importance to surgeons because the mucosa above the line is supplied by nerves from the autonomic system which supply all the viscera. It can be operated on or injected without causing pain. Below the dentate line the skin is innervated by ordinary peripheral nerves and any injury is very painful.

Just above the dentate line the submucosa is a little thicker and more vascular. These areas of thickening are called the anal cushions.

The lymphatic drainage of the rectum is into the lymph nodes of the pelvis and abdomen but the anal canal drains into lymph nodes in the groin which are called the inguinal nodes. Cancer of the anal canal may spread by these lymphatic vessels to the inguinal lymph nodes.

Examination of the Anal Canal

The term piles is synonymous with internal haemorrhoids. Patients with any abnormality of the anus tend to say they have piles and careful examination is needed to make an exact diagnosis. All doctors and nurses need to remember constantly that patients are greatly embarrassed when talking about anal troubles and even more troubled by examination. They should be treated with the utmost tact and covered as much as possible consistent with the examination. Most surgeons examine the anus with the patient in the left lateral position. The hips and knees are well flexed and the shoulder tilted forwards from the exact lateral position. The surgeon will need to inspect the anus in a good light and the fibre-light cable is useful for this purpose. Following this he will make a digital examination of the rectum using a disposable glove well lubricated with KY jelly. At all times the surgeon must tell the patient what he is about to do so that his confidence is not lost. Next follows examination of the anal canal and lower end of the rectum with a steel proctoscope (Fig. 58). This instrument is cold and should be warmed by placing it in warm water. A cold instrument causes unnecessary discomfort and also spasm of the sphincter. The proctoscope is a steel cylinder or speculum with an inner removable part called the obturator. When the instrument has been passed into the rectum the obturator is removed and the fibre-light cable fixed to the proctoscope.

Internal Haemorrhoids

The condition of internal haemorrhoids results from enlargement of the vascular anal cushions. These in no way resemble varicose veins but venous obstruction such as results from pregnancy and straining because of constipation causes engorgement and enlargement of the anal cushions.

Haemorrhoids which arise during pregnancy usually regress completely after delivery.

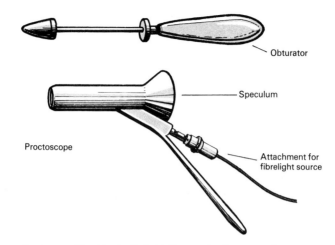

Proctoscope. The obturator fits inside the speculum for easy passing and is removed when the instrument is in the rectum

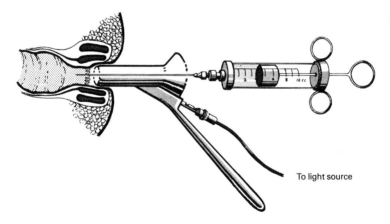

Fig 58 Proctoscope being used for the injection of haemorrhoids with Gabriel's needle and syringe

It is customary to describe three degrees of haemorrhoids:

First degree haemorrhoids are inside the anus and the patient complains of bleeding with the stool.

Second degree haemorrhoids have grown to a considerable size so that in addition to bleeding the patient notices that the haemorrhoid prolapses outside the anus on defaecation but returns easily with a little pressure.

Third degree haemorrhoids are so large that they are permanently prolapsed.

Uncomplicated haemorrhoids are painless and if the patient is complaining of pain the haemorrhoid must be strangulated and thrombosed. In this condition the soft haemorrhoid is converted to a hard lump because of thrombosis of the blood in its veins. Such a lump stretches the skin and causes considerable pain. In addition, because the lump is solid it will not reduce into the anal canal and remains as an anal lump. Haemorrhoids can be seen and diagnosed on proctoscopy or by simple inspection if they are prolapsed.

Treatment of Internal Haemorrhoids

1   *Injection with 5% phenol in oil* (Fig. 58)

Injections are suitable for first and early second degree haemorrhoids. The injection is given into the tissue at the upper part of the haemorrhoid with the object of causing fibrosis which will make the haemorrhoid contract. It is not an intravenous injection. The oily solution is very viscous and considerable pressure is needed to inject the haemorrhoid. A special syringe called a Gabriel syringe is used which has a locking device to prevent the needle separating from the syringe during the injection. The needles have to be long enough to pass through the proctoscope and they have a guard about 1 cm from the tip to prevent too deep penetration of the needle. The injection is above the dentate line of the anal canal and is entirely painless. It is better to tell the patient after he has been given the injection as nobody believes that an injection here will be painless.

2   *Elastic Bands*

In this form of treatment elastic bands are placed on the haemorrhoid using a special instrument. Access is again secured with a proctoscope. It is suitable for the same type of case as might be treated with injections and the choice remains with the surgeon who may prefer one technique or the other. Provided the bands are placed above the dentate line the treatment is painless. As with injections this treatment is given in the outpatient clinic.

3   *Cryosurgery*

Cryosurgery may be used for all types of haemorrhoids but the cryoprobe must be kept above the dentate line if it is to be painless.

The cryoprobe is an instrument which reaches a low temperature as a result of the expansion of a gas. The probe is connected to a cylinder of nitrous oxide and held against the haemorrhoid for two or three minutes. A large ice crystal forms during the treatment and causes necrosis of the haemorrhoid. Cryosurgery is used for haemorrhoids too large for treatment by injection or elastic bands. It can be done with a local or general anaesthetic. A plastic non-conductor speculum is used as a steel proctoscope would get very cold and possibly cause extensive mucosal necrosis.

The treatment is done as a day case but the patient is told to expect a slight discharge from the anus for a few days. He should be given Isogel to take as a stool softener for about a week.

Operative Treatment of Haemorrhoids

Most patients have heard that this operation can be very painful and many dread having to undergo haemorrhoidectomy. The operation is now less often performed because of the development of new techniques which are easier and less painful. However, it is still done for third degree haemorrhoids, i.e. those which are large, prolapse easily, and do not return inside the anal canal without external pressure.

Preoperative Management

The whole management of haemorrhoidectomy has to be carried out with the utmost tact. Also the patient is likely to be fearful of postoperative pain. This should not be unduly minimised and the best attitude which the nurse can take is to say that pain can be relieved with suitable drugs. Dishonesty, even when well intentioned, has no place in medical care. If the patient is told not to worry and that the operation will be painless he will never believe the profession again if he suffers pain after the operation.

The anal area has considerable resistance to bacterial invasion and antibacterial agents are not necessary. Most surgeons ask for the distal colon to be emptied before the operation with a phosphate enema the night before and another about 3 hours before the operation. Vague instructions from the doctor to give an enema are sometimes followed by an enema on the night before the operation. If an enema is not given just before, the rectum may easily have refilled. If only one enema is given it is better that it should be immediately preoperative.

The worst pain following haemorrhoidectomy occurs at the time of the first bowel action after the operation. To minimise this the patient should be given a stool softener such as Isogel beginning on the night before the operation.

It is unnecessary to shave more than the immediate perianal area.

The Operation

Various types of anaesthetic may be given—general, epidural and even local infiltration.

The operation consists of a simple removal of the haemorrhoids which are ligatured with catgut or silk and then excised. The ligatures are usually left long and hang out of the anus. The wound is not sutured following excision because faeces would infect a sutured wound. With the wound left open to granulate and then to close by growth of skin from the edges, infection is superficial and within a few days the wounds look pink and uninfected. At the end of the operation some surgeons leave a small vaseline gauze pack in the anal canal to control bleeding. A dressing is placed over the perineum and kept in place with a T-bandage. A sanitary towel also provides a good and convenient dressing to absorb bleeding from the excisions.

Postoperative Care

Haemorrhoidectomy is a painful operation and the first bowel action is usually difficult and painful. Analgesics are used freely but morphine derivatives are best avoided as they cause constipation and make the first bowel action more difficult. A stool softener such as Isogel is given nightly and if the bowels are not open spontaneously by the second day an aperient such as Dulcolax is given on the second postoperative evening.

The patient is sat in a hot bath or on a bidet from the first morning and at the first bath the opportunity is taken to remove the pack. The patient may be allowed to remove this himself in the bath if he wishes but patients and nurses should know that the long sutures are to be left to separate spontaneously. This usually happens on about the 7th to the 10th day according to the size of the haemorrhoids. The hot bathing has two effects. The first is that it is an easy and relatively painless way of cleaning the area after bowel actions. The second is that immersion in hot water relaxes spasm in the anal sphincter muscle which is the cause of postoperative pain. The patient should be allowed three or four baths daily and analgesia achieved in this way is more effective than the use of oral analgesics. The economic value of a bidet is obvious as it requires only a fraction of the quantity of hot water.

Most surgeons do not ask for any special dietary restrictions.

After each bowel action the wound area is cleaned with hot water in the bath or on the bidet and a simple sterile gauze or eusol dressing applied and kept in place with a T-bandage or tight pants.

Discharge is usually about the 6th or 7th day. The patient must not be allowed home until the bowel action has returned to normal. Some surgeons like to keep the patient in hospital until the ligatures have separated as separation is sometimes accompanied by some bleeding. The excision wounds may not be completely healed for up to 6 or 8 weeks.

Complications of Haemorrhoidectomy

The operation is surprisingly free from complications and those which are described are rare.

Haemorrhage

This may occur soon after return to the ward following the operation and is an example of primary haemorrhage. Although rare it can be very dramatic and blood loss into the bed considerable. In addition to the routine postoperative observations of pulse rate and blood pressure it is wise to take a look under the sheets from time to time within the first few hours to see that no bleeding is taking place. Primary bleeding may stop spontaneously but the medical staff must be alerted and in some cases the surgeon will take the patient back to the operating theatre to stop the bleeding.

Secondary haemorrhage occurs later but is rarely significant. Some bleeding often occurs when the ligatures separate.

Stricture of the Anus

If too much skin has been removed at the time of the operation a fibrous stricture may occur as healing takes place. Many surgeons do a rectal examination before the patient is discharged to assess the amount of fibrosis developing after the operation. Rectal examination also discloses faecal impaction which must be dealt with before discharge if it is present.

Retention of Urine

Although this is not solely a complication of haemorrhoidectomy it is quite a common problem especially in men. Simple measures are usually sufficient to overcome retention, which is due to spasm in the bladder sphincter associated with spasm in the anal sphincter. The patient may be able to pass urine if he is allowed to stand in privacy. If there is a risk that he might faint and fall he can be advised to pass urine in the sitting position or sitting on the bidet with hot water may relax the sphincter and enable him to pass urine.

Complications of Haemorrhoids

The only complication of haemorrhoids is thrombosis. When a haemorrhoid prolapses outside the anus it may be strangulated by a tight anal sphincter which prevents its re-entry inside the anus. The blood in the haemorrhoid soon thromboses converting the soft easily reducible haemorrhoid into a solid mass which cannot be reduced. The patient is aware of a tender lump at the anus which makes sitting and defaecation very painful. When this complication occurs the general public diagnose 'an attack of piles'. If nothing is done the thrombus is gradually replaced by fibrous tissue and over a period of about 10 to 14 days the haemorrhoid reduces in size until it is reduced to a small tag of skin at the anus. Following an attack of strangulation and thrombosis the patient may notice a considerable improvement in the symptoms of his haemorrhoids which may no longer be large enough to prolapse.

The condition is easily diagnosed by inspection of the anus. Proctoscopy is generally not performed at this stage but delayed until the acute phase has subsided. Although some surgeons advise excision in the acute phase most leave the strangulation to settle down and reassess the haemorrhoids by proctoscopy after two to three weeks. Patients with an acute attack of 'piles' are nursed with the foot of the bed elevated. Pain is relieved with drugs and the local application of cold compresses which help to reduce swelling.

Anal Fissure (Fig. 59)

An anal fissure is a crack which forms at the anal verge and is usually attributed to the passage of a hard motion. In most cases there is no special underlying cause but in a few cases it is associated with Crohn's disease of the intestine.

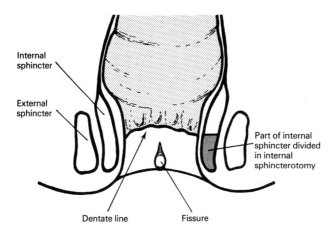

Internal sphincter

External sphincter

Part of internal sphincter divided in internal sphincterotomy

Dentate line   Fissure

Fig 59   Anal fissure

The outstanding clinical feature of an anal fissure is great pain on defaecation and for up to two hours afterwards. The motion may be streaked with blood but this is not a significant feature. In some patients a fissure heals spontaneously but in many it becomes chronic and the patient continues to have great pain until relieved by surgical intervention.

Examination is difficult and should initially be confined to inspection. If the anal skin is separated it is possible to see the fissure which is usually but not always located posteriorly. Most surgeons do not proceed to rectal examination let alone proctoscopy if a fissure is seen as it causes great pain. Instead the patient is admitted urgently for examination under an anaesthetic. In a few middle-aged patients this shows a cancer of the anal canal to be the cause of the symptoms.

Treatment

It is believed that spasm in the anal sphincter prevents healing. Certainly the sphincter is in spasm as is shown by any attempt at rectal examination. Treatment is aimed at preventing spasm in the sphincter muscle so allowing the fissure to heal. One way of achieving this is to stretch the anal muscle under a general anaesthetic. This cures about 80 % of patients. Those which recur are treated by internal sphincterotomy.

Internal Sphincterotomy.   In this operation an incision, about 2 cm in length, is made at the side of the anus and through this incision the lower part of the internal sphincter, up to the level of the dentate line, is divided with scissors. The incision is usually closed with catgut sutures.

There is no preoperative preparation other than the use of a stool softener such as Isogel. Attempts at enemas or washouts are too painful and, as the operation is outside the anus, unnecessary. A very local shave may be possible but if the anal spasm prevents access this can easily be done in the operating theatre. A sphincterotomy can be done under local, caudal or general anaesthetic. Anal dilatation is done on an outpatient basis. Internal sphincterotomy can also be done as an outpatient procedure but if beds allow it many surgeons prefer to keep the patient in for 24 hours. There is no special after-treatment and relief from pain is usually immediate and dramatic. The catgut sutures are allowed to separate spontaneously.

Perianal Haematoma (Fig. 60)

This is sometimes called an external pile or haemorrhoid. It is a condition which tends to occur in young adults and comprises a perianal lump which is tense, blue and painful. It is caused by a spontaneous haemorrhage from a superficial vein and is in fact a localised collection of blood or haematoma, which is painful and tender because it is under some tension.

If left alone a haematoma will absorb in about 10 days leaving little sign except perhaps a small tag of excess skin over the site of the lump. As an alternative the haematoma can be evacuated under local anaesthetic in the outpatient department. Anal wounds are usually left open to heal by granulation and a small clean or eusol dressing,

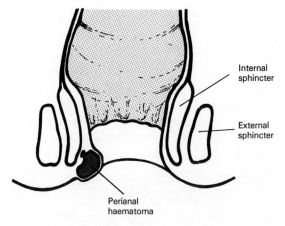

Internal
sphincter

External
sphincter

Perianal
haematoma

Fig 60   A perianal haematoma resulting from bleeding from a small vein

kept in place by tight pants, will be necessary until the wound is healed. Bathing after bowel action helps to keep the wound clean.

Anorectal Abscess (Fig. 61)

The fatty spaces adjacent to the anal canal and the lower rectum are subject to infections leading to abscess formation. The exact way in which the infection begins is subject to discussion but one theory is that it begins as an infection in the anal glands which lie between the sphincters and which discharge into the anal canal. Bacterial infection from the anal canal reaches the intersphincteric region along the duct of an anal gland.

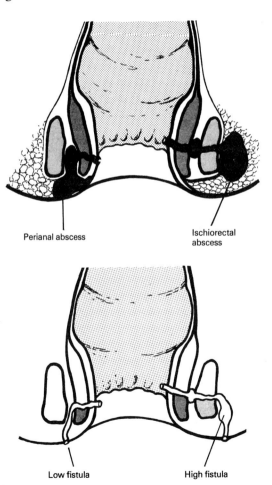

Fig 61 Anal abscess and fistula

The two common sites for infection are the perianal and the ischiorectal spaces. Once infection is established the patient complains of severe and continuous pain in the rectum and adjacent to the anus. A perianal abscess causes localised swelling and tenderness but the ischiorectal abscess does not cause swelling in the early stages as it is deeply placed. This may account for the late diagnosis in some cases but the tender swelling is easily felt if the doctor does a rectal examination.

If a perirectal abscess is left to follow a natural course it will eventually discharge into the anal canal or through the perianal skin or in both directions about the same time (Fig. 61). If the abscess bursts into the anal canal as well as to the skin surface a granulation lined tube is created connecting the anal canal with the skin. Such a tube is called a fistula. Although this may seem to heal it gets reinfected from the anal canal causing recurrent perianal abscesses. A granulation lined tube resulting from an abscess and opening in only one direction is called a sinus. Fistulae and sinuses occur in many parts of the body.

Treatment of Anorectal Abscess

Although antibiotic treatment may be given it is important to open an abscess as early as possible before it bursts into the anal canal forming a fistula. There is no special preoperative management but the patient is taken to the operating theatre as soon as convenient and the abscess incised through an incision in the perianal skin. The object is to promote healing from the depth rather than early closure of the skin cover which will result in recurrence of the abscess. With this object in mind the surgeon will often leave in a corrugated drain secured with a suture and also a length of gauze soaked in a mixture of eusol and paraffin. The addition of paraffin to eusol makes it easier and less painful to remove. These wounds are often challenging as it is necessary to repack the wound daily to promote healing from the base. This means that the pack must be accurately placed but not so tightly as to interfere with the drainage of pus.

Treatment of Anorectal Fistula

Operations for fistula are as old as history and King Louis XIV of France is one of many said to have had such an operation. The principle is that the fistula will only heal if it is opened from end to end and the wound converted to a saucer shape by excision of tissue at the edges. To accomplish this the surgeon usually has to cut through parts of both anal sphincters at the level at which the fistula passes through. Division of a small part of the anal sphincter has no effect on anal continence. In dealing with a high fistula it may be necessary to divide sufficient muscle to interfere with normal continence. Luckily most fistulae are low and no interference with continence is to be expected.

The second effect of an operation for fistula is that a very large wound is left which will be difficult to handle and will take many weeks to heal. The surgeon's difficulties are increased by the fact that in many cases the fistula is not simply a straight track but has branches, all of which have to be opened into the same final wound. Of course the patient does not need to stay in hospital until the wound is completely healed but a simple fistula wound will not be healed inside four weeks and a wound resulting from an operation on a complicated fistula may take up to three months to heal.

Preoperative treatment consists in getting the colon and rectum as empty as possible. It is obvious that it will be better for the patient if his bowels are not open for several days after the operation so that the large wound has a chance to cover with granulation tissue which is an effective natural barrier against the entry of infection.

Postoperative treatment is mainly directed to the care of the large open wound. The principle is the same as for wounds following incision of an anorectal abscess but the wound following a fistula operation tends to be much larger. At the end of the operation the wound is lightly packed with gauze soaked in eusol or eusol and paraffin and this is kept in position with a T-bandage. In difficult cases the first dressing is done after 4 or 5 days and then in the operating theatre under an anaesthetic. In dealing with smaller wounds and for subsequent dressings the use of Entonox inhalation is a useful way of minimising pain. In dealing with the actual dressing the object is to repack lightly so that drainage can still take place but the packing is to the edge of the wound to discourage closure from the edges and encourage healing from the depth in the first place.

Retention of urine may be a problem and if the patient is having difficulty it may be easier for him to have an indwelling catheter for a week or so.

Prolapse of the Rectum (Fig. 62)

Prolapse of the rectum generally occurs in elderly people in whom the muscles of the pelvic floor and anus are weak allowing the rectum to prolapse out through the anus.

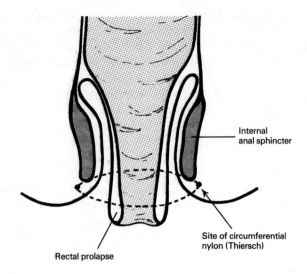

Fig 62   Rectal prolapse

Rectal prolapse also occurs in infants but this is an entirely different condition which does not require surgical treatment because of natural remission.

Patients with prolapse are usually greatly troubled by the condition. The rectum prolapses with defaecation and also in some patients spontaneously while walking about. The mass of rectum outside the anus is not painful but it is very uncomfortable and may bleed. A more troublesome complication is incontinence. This is partly due to the poor anal sphincter muscles but it is also caused by the act of prolapse. If there are faeces in the rectum these are carried outside when the rectum prolapses.

A great many operations have been used in the treatment of rectal prolapse. In medical care it is important to avoid diarrhoea and a constipating drug such as codeine phosphate may be necessary. The operations are generally divided into those performed from above and those performed from below.

Thiersch Operation

Thiersch introduced the idea of a suture encircling the anus as long ago as 1891 when he used a length of silver wire (Fig. 62). The operation fell into disuse until the 1950s when it was reintroduced. Later nylon was used in place of wire. The obvious benefit of the operation is its simplicity and safety in a patient who is often old and frail. Unfortunately the operation has not been very successful and is not in very common use at present. If the nylon suture is tied too tightly the patient has difficulty with bowel action and if it is too loose the rectum continues to prolapse. However, it is still used in some very frail patients.

Ivalon Sponge Repair

The operations from above are performed through an abdominal incision. In these the rectum is freed from the surrounding structures. Some surgeons try to repair the muscles of the pelvic floor but this is a difficult task. Wells, in Liverpool in 1955, described the use of a piece of Ivalon (polyvinyl alcohol) which was wrapped round the rectum. This plastic foreign body induced adhesions so fixing the rectum to the front of the sacrum and preventing prolapse.

Le Haut Operation

Probably the simplest operation from above is to mobilise the rectum and to prevent prolapse by fixing it in the anterior abdominal wall. This is called Le Haut's operation and it enjoys some popularity at the present time.

Postoperative Care

There is no specific postoperative care except the usual treatment required after any laparotomy. As no resection has been done the course is usually smooth. It is unwise for the patient to strain when passing a stool until the rectum has become fixed by fibrous tissue so a stool softener such as Isogel should be given.

20

Hernia

A hernia is defined as a bulge or protusion of part of the contents of a cavity through an orifice, the hernial orifice, to the tissues outside the cavity.

Groin Hernia

There are two types of hernia in the groin. One is called a femoral hernia because it passes through the femoral canal which is a weak area leading from the abdomen to the thigh. A femoral hernia presents as a lump in the thigh just below the groin.

The second type of hernia is called an inguinal hernia. One type of inguinal hernia is called a direct inguinal hernia. This is a bulge of the rather weak part of the abdominal wall just above the groin. It presents as a lump in this position. The second type of inguinal hernia is called an indirect inguinal hernia because it takes a slanting, indirect course through the abdominal wall instead of the direct bulge forward of the direct inguinal hernia.

The spermatic cord consists of the vas deferens which carries sperm from the testis and the artery and veins carrying testicular blood. The spermatic cord leaves the abdomen through an opening called the internal inguinal ring which allows the cord to enter the abdominal wall between the deep and superficial muscles. It passes medially for about two inches in this layer and then completes its transit through the abdominal wall at the external ring. The testis develops at the back of the abdomen and migrates or descends to its adult position just before birth. In doing so it carries a projection from the peritoneal cavity which is shaped like the finger of a glove. This extension from the peritoneal cavity normally closes in infancy but if it persists it is called a hernial sac. The walls of the sac may remain stuck together but as a result of straining, which raises the intra-abdominal pressure, some part of the abdominal contents eventually pass into the sac producing a lump just above the groin which is called an indirect inguinal hernia.

Although there is an anatomical distinction it is sometimes difficult for a surgeon to decide if a particular hernia is of the direct or indirect type by clinical examination. Femoral hernia and indirect inguinal hernias are subject to a serious complication called strangulation, so that it is usual to recommend operative repair of all groin hernias to avoid this complication.

When intestine or fat pass through a hernial orifice a bulge results which can be made to disappear if the patient lies down and applies some pressure over the lump, so reducing the contents back into the abdominal cavity. If the contents are compressed at the hernial orifice or ring the blood supply to the hernial contents are cut off and after some hours become gangrenous. This is called strangulation.

Treatment of Hernia

The only satisfactory treatment of a hernia is an operative repair. Some patients fear surgery and others are not fit for an operation under a general anaesthetic. For these patients a truss may be prescribed. This consists of a pad which is held over the hernial orifice by a metal spring which encircles the trunk and a strap which passes between the legs to prevent the truss from riding up. Not only is a truss uncomfortable but it rarely keeps the hernia reduced; strangulatation can occur while the patient is wearing it. Now that hernias can be operated on under local anaesthetic a truss is very rarely the correct treatment.

Operations for Groin Hernia

The principle of the operation is to excise the hernia sac and to repair the area with nylon. This may be done under general or local anaesthetic. If the operation is done under a general anaesthetic the patient will generally be kept in hospital overnight and discharged the following day but some surgeons prefer to keep patients in hospital for a few days.

Hernia Repair under Local Anaesthetic

If the repair is done under local anaesthetic the whole procedure can be carried out as an outpatient procedure. However, it is essential to liaise fully with the community nursing service if this technique is to be used. The patient is advised that he may have breakfast and is admitted to the day surgery unit about $1\frac{1}{2}$ hours before the time scheduled for the operation. A premedication such as Omnopon and Fentazin may be given but many surgeons prefer to do this operation without premedication. The surgeon gives the local anaesthetic and does exactly the same operation as would be done under a general anaesthetic. During the operation a screen is placed so that the patient cannot see the operation and a nurse sits with him. The object of this is to give confidence and to talk to him so distracting him from the operation. Any subject can be discussed but it is wise to avoid asking the patient if he is feeling pain as this may lead to loss of confidence. At the end of the operation the patient dresses and is discharged immediately. It is important for him to leave at once so that he reaches home before the effects of the local anaesthetic wear off. Arrangements are made for visits from the community nurse on the evening of the operation and again to remove the sutures. The patient is given a small supply of pain relieving drugs. Complications are very unusual and probably less than when a general anaesthetic is used.

Although this technique is not yet used in many centres it is so successful and economical that it seems likely to become much more popular in the next ten years.

Postoperative Care

Patients are told not to do any heavy lifting following a hernia operation as this will put strain on the repair and possibly lead to recurrence. Free movement is encouraged and the patient may walk as much as he wishes from the day following the operation. Recurrence is rare now that the repair is done with strong and nonabsorbable material such as nylon and the period off heavy work is less than formerly. A patient should be able to return to any work in two months.

Strangulated Hernia

Sometimes a hernia cannot be replaced because of adhesion of the contents to the sac. This is called an irreducible hernia and is not a serious complication. In other cases the hernia is so constricted at the hernial orifice that the bowel lumen is closed causing intestinal obstruction and the blood supply of the intestine is also cut off. This is a most serious condition called strangulation and the intestine in the sac will die. There is secondary infection of the dead tissue with intestinal organisms and the result is black putrefying intestine which is called gangrene.

A strangulated hernia is an acute surgical emergency. The patient will need preoperative treatment like any other case of intestinal obstruction. In particular he will need a gastric tube to aspirate gastric contents to prevent vomiting and also an intravenous infusion of fluid to replace that lost in the dilated, obstructed intestine and also by vomiting. Antibiotics are also given to control bacterial invasion of the tissues and blood stream from the gangrenous tissue.

The first part of the operation is to relieve the constricting ring and to inspect the strangulated intestine. If the surgeon judges that it is not viable he will remove it. The operation is completed by removal of the hernial sac and repair with nylon.

Umbilical Hernia

Two types of hernia occur at the umbilicus:

1 **Umbilical hernia** which is a defect in the umbilical scar. This type of hernia is seen in infancy and shows a natural tendency to regression. Trusses or supports are unnecessary as the hernia causes no symptoms and strangulation is unknown. If the hernia is still present by the age of five years it is repaired under a general anaesthetic. This operation is best done as an outpatient procedure.

2 **Paraumbilical hernia** is an aquired hernia which occurs in middle aged and obese people. It is above or below the umbilicus and bulges into it. These hernias can reach a large size and there is also a possibility of strangulation of small intestine which is contained in the sac. Surgical treatment is usually advised after a period of dieting to achieve weight loss. In modern surgery the umbilicus is always preserved.

Incisional Hernia

Any incision on the anterior abdominal wall may break down and form a hernia many years later. The incisional hernia may reach a large size and is a cosmetic problem, particularly in women. There is also a danger of strangulation.

The choice of treatment lies between the use of an abdominal corset to reduce and support the hernia and operative repair. A corset is used if the patient is unfit for surgery or grossly obese. There is a high recurrence rate following repair of an incisional hernia in an obese patient and operation should be deferred while the patient loses weight. Operative repair consists of excising the hernia sac and repairing the abdominal wall to restore the normal anatomy.

21

The Skin

The skin encloses and protects the body. It is richly supplied with sensory nerves and any injury to the skin is painful.

The skin is made of two distinct parts. The deep part or dermis is a fibroelastic layer containing the sweat glands and the hair follicles or roots. The sweat which is made in the glands reaches the surface of the skin through tiny sweat ducts. As it evaporates it has the effect of cooling the body.

The superficial part of the skin is called the epidermis and is made of epithelial cells. A layer of cells at the base of the epidermis is called the basal layer. These cells constantly divide to produce more skin cells which migrate to the surface as more cells are produced by the basal layer. When the cells reach the surface they flake off.

Scattered among the basal layer of cells there are some cells called melanocytes which are stimulated by sunlight to produce a brown pigment called melanin.

Skin Cysts

The sebaceous cyst or wen is a common cyst in the skin. It may arise as a retention cyst caused by obstruction of the duct of a sebaceous gland. In other cases it is an epidermoid cyst lined with typical skin. Sometimes a sebaceous cyst becomes infected and forms an abscess. The treatment is excision under local anaesthetic.

Angiomas

Angiomas are malformations of blood vessels. They are usually birthmarks or appear soon after birth. The port wine stain is a diffuse area of wine coloured staining in the skin which is present at birth. It is unfortunate that there is no effective treatment because the face and neck are often affected.

The strawberry naevus or angioma usually appears soon after birth and has the colour and appearance of a strawberry. It grows with the child and then regresses and disappears about the age of five years. It is important to avoid treatment as natural regression leaves no scar and all forms of intervention give an ultimately less good result.

Tumours of the Skin

Most people have some benign tumours of the skin. Warts are common especially around the neck and are produced by viruses. A mole is a brown skin tumour which arises from the melanocytes. It is often a malformation and is seen in childhood. Most people have a number of moles. Another name for a mole is a naevus. Treatment is not usually necessary.

There are three malignant tumours of the skin:

1   Epithelioma

Epithelioma or carcinoma of the skin may occur anywhere but in the elderly it is inclined to occur on exposed parts. It may also complicate a long standing venous ulcer of the leg. Epithelioma spreads locally and also through the lymphatic vessels to the lymph nodes. These tumours are sensitive to radiation and treatment may be by local excision or radiotherapy. Secondary nodes are usually treated by excision.

2   Basal Cell Carcinoma or Rodent Ulcer

This tumour is unique in having locally invasive qualities but never spreading by the lymph or blood vessels. Eighty percent of basal tumours occur on the face and there is no doubt that sunlight is an aetiological factor. White skinned Europeans who have emigrated to Australia show a high incidence of multiple basal cell tumours because of the increased exposure to sunlight.

The basal cell carcinoma is highly sensitive to radiotherapy which is the standard treatment.

3   Malignant Melanoma

Malignant melanoma arises in the melanocytes of the skin. Some tumours arise in a pre-existing benign melanoma or mole. The transformation to malignancy is sometimes stimulated by trauma and this includes an ill-advised local removal for cosmetic reasons.

Melanomata are variable in their malignancy but some are extremely dangerous. They are all completely resistant to radiotherapy and cure depends on surgical removal. The tumour spreads locally and there is sometimes a halo of pigment around the tumour. The main spread is through the lymph vessels but blood stream spread is also common in the later stages. The treatment is very wide local excision, often combined with resection of the lymphatic nodes. A skin graft is usually necessary to close the defect following excision.

22

The Surgery of Trauma

Primary Management of a Major Accident

When a patient is admitted to the accident department the doctor's first task is to make a diagnosis. However, a patient with multiple injuries may be so critically ill that the first priority is to save life and to defer making a diagnosis until steps have been taken to correct life-threatening problems and to stabilise the general condition.

The two critical problems are hypovolaemic shock resulting from blood loss and an obstructed airway and each of these can cause death:

1   The common cause of obstruction of the airway in an unconscious patient is closure of the pharynx by the back of the tongue, which falls backwards. This can often be remedied by pulling the jaw forwards with a finger behind each angle of the jaw. This is effective because the tongue is attached to the back of the jaw and the tongue comes forward clearing the pharynx when the jaw is pulled forward. In some patients vomit is responsible for obstructing the airway. Vomit can be removed with a sucker or with the fingers. A simple airway can be inserted to maintain the airway (Fig. 63). Another technique is to put the patient in the semiprone position so that the tongue falls forwards instead of back, so clearing the airway. This is particularly useful in an emergency and for transporting the patient. If the airway continues to be obstructed or if breathing is ineffectual the patient is intubated. This means that a tube is passed into the trachea and used to provide air directly into the trachea (Fig. 63). If the patient's own breathing is inadequate the lungs can be inflated and deflated by connecting the tube to a machine which delivers air or oxygen under sufficient pressure to inflate the lung. After each inflation the machine removes the pressure and the lungs deflate. Respiration removes carbon dioxide from the blood and provides a supply of oxygen. Inadequate breathing causes a fall in the oxygen in the blood (anoxia) and rise in carbon dioxide (hyper-capnia). If this is prolonged it may cause irreversible damage to the brain and kidneys.

2   In all cases in which the blood pressure is low it is likely that the cause is blood loss causing hypovolaemic shock. Such blood loss cannot be the result of a brain injury because of the limited space inside the skull, but considerable blood loss can result from a scalp

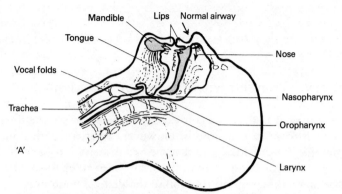

An unconscious patient in the supine position. Air enters the nostril and passes through the nose, the nasopharynx and oropharynx. It then goes forward to enter the larynx, passing the vocal folds to enter the trachea. In this position the tongue is seen to drop back so occluding the oropharynx. The diagram shows how the tongue is attached to the back of the jaw

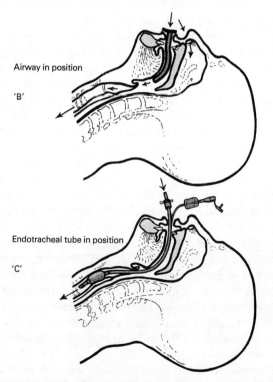

Fig 63 Treatment of airway obstruction

injury. In many cases the blood loss is caused by an injury in another part of the body. For example, a great deal of blood can be lost into the pleural cavity in complicated fractures of the ribs and trauma to the abdomen may cause rupture of the liver or spleen which results in blood loss into the peritoneal cavity. This is a large space and can accommodate a large volume of blood. Major fractures such as a fracture of the femur can cause a haematoma in the leg which may be filled with as much as a litre of blood. Whatever the cause of the blood loss the blood volume must be increased urgently by transfusion of blood or other fluid, so restoring the circulation to the brain and kidneys. It is unusual to see external arterial bleeding but if this is present it can be stopped by applying strong local pressure over the bleeding point. A tourniquet above the bleeding point is rarely necessary. If one is used, the pressure in the cuff must be above arterial pressure.

Head Injuries

Head injuries account for about half the deaths caused by road accidents and a quarter of deaths due to all kinds of trauma. A head injury may be isolated but in many cases the clinical situation is complicated by multiple injuries.

Anatomy and Pathology

The brain is encased in the skull which affords protection against trauma. It is possible to sustain severe brain damage without a fracture of the skull, but a fracture is present in about 80 % of cases of head injury in which there is severe brain damage.

Primary brain damage occurs at the time of the injury. There may be areas of haemorrhage (contusions) in the brain and diffuse injury to the nerve fibres in the white matter of the brain resulting from violent movement of the brain inside the skull. In minor trauma to the head the cerebrospinal fluid, which lies between the brain and the skull, cushions the brain and protects it. The degree of brain damage varies from case to case but diffuse damage causes unconsciousness which may vary in depth and also in duration. A short period of unconsciousness used to be called concussion.

Secondary brain damage may be caused by the development of a localised haematoma within the skull as a result of continued bleeding from an injured artery or vein. The skull is an unyielding box encasing the brain so that when a haematoma forms within the skull it inevitably compresses the brain. A thick membrane called the tentorium cerebelli lies across the inside of the skull (Fig. 64). The cerebral hemispheres are above the tentorium and the cerebellum and medulla are below. A haematoma which forms above the tentorium will have the additional affect of pressing a part of the cerebral hemisphere down through the tentorium where it causes pressure on

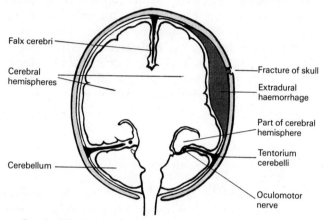

Falx cerebri

Cerebral hemispheres

Cerebellum

Fracture of skull

Extradural haemorrhage

Part of cerebral hemisphere

Tentorium cerebelli

Oculomotor nerve

Extradural haemorrhage shown in a coronal section of the skull *i.e.* one running from one ear to the other

Extradural haematoma compressing the brain and pushing part of one cerebral hemisphere through the opening in the tentorium cerebelli where it presses upon the oculomotor nerve

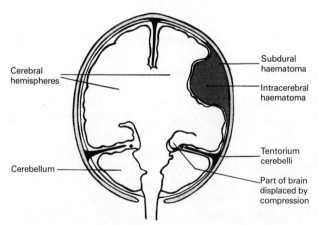

Cerebral hemispheres

Cerebellum

Subdural haematoma

Intracerebral haematoma

Tentorium cerebelli

Part of brain displaced by compression

Coronal section of the brain showing intradural haematoma which is partly subdural and partly intracerebral. There is compression of the brain and actual brain trauma

Fig 64   Intracranial haemorrhage

a nerve called the oculomotor nerve, because it controls some of the muscles which move the eye on the same side and also controls the size of the pupil. Pressure on this nerve interferes with its function and causes characteristic eye signs.

Brain damage is compounded by lack of oxygen (anoxia). This may be due to interference with breathing caused by a chest injury or by poor circulation resulting from haemorrhage. Restoration of the circulating blood volume and improvement of breathing will help to restore brain function.

Early Monitoring and Management of a Patient with a Head Injury

Although the patient is unconscious it must never be forgotten that he is a person who will hopefully, in time, recover consciousness. Every possible care is to be given to his management and, as consciousness returns, to his comfort. It is also a most stressful time for the relatives who must be kept informed of the patient's progress and be given every facility to be with their loved one as much as possible. Intensive care wards need comfortable and cheerfully furnished rooms for anxious waiting relatives. Relatives should also be able to spend the night in the hospital when the patient's condition is particularly serious.

When a patient is unconscious there are two distinct aims of medical care. The first is to set up life support systems which have already been described and which ensure that respiration and blood circulation are maintained. The second aim is to collect regular data on which his condition and progress can be assessed. This system of data collection at regular intervals is called monitoring.

1 Circulatory Monitoring

These measurements consist of the pulse rate, blood pressure and central venous pressure.

2 Urinary Output

Measurement of the urinary output is an indication of renal function and can be readily assessed only if a catheter is placed in the bladder so that the production of urine can be measured at regular intervals and not be subject to the time intervals of normal micturition. Unconscious patients are incontinent of urine and the catheter has the added advantage that the urine is not passed into the bed so making pressure necrosis more likely.

3   Blood Gases

Air enters and leaves the body through the air passages. As these get smaller in the lungs they are first called bronchi and then bronchioles. At the end of the smallest bronchiole there is a tiny sac called an alveolus which has a capillary blood vessel in its wall. Air which is inspired reaches the alveolus and oxygen passes from the air through the wall of the alveolus and capillary to enter the blood. Carbon dioxide leaves the blood and enters the air in the alveolus at the same time and is removed in expiration.

The exchange of oxygen and carbon dioxide depends on normal respiratory function.

Patients who are suspected of having inadequate lung function for any reason are given oxygen through a mask at a rate of about 4 litres a minute.

Blood gas analysis is used to confirm the adequacy of normal respiration and any oxygen supplement which may be given.

For this test blood is taken from an artery. The radial artery at the wrist is often used but if the patient is collapsed, puncture of a small artery will be difficult and a larger artery such as the femoral may be used. A small quantity of heparin is first sucked into the syringe and then squirted out to leave only a trace in the syringe. After collection of the arterial blood, care is taken to see that there is no air in the syringe because this would be a source of extra oxygen to the blood. As soon as the needle is removed the syringe is capped to prevent contamination of the specimen with oxygen from the air. The blood gases are estimated on a machine and the test should be done as quickly as possible. If the specimen has to be transported far it should be immersed in ice.

The results are expressed as Pao_2 or $Paco_2$ where 'P' stands for pressure, 'a' for artery and 'o_2' and 'co_2' for oxygen and carbon dioxide. Until recently the pressure of a gas was expressed in mm of mercury and the normal Pao_2 was 100 mm of mercury. In the new SI units gas pressure is expressed in a unit which is called a kilopascal (kPa) and the equivalent to 100 mm of mercury is 13 kPa. If the arterial oxygen is found to be low it can be corrected in a variety of ways, including inhalation of oxygen and the use of assisted respiration.

4 Hydration and Feeding

During the early phase of management, an intravenous infusion is the best route for continued hydration. If the patient remains unconscious for more than three days he can be given intravenous feeding, but it is safer and easier to give food through an intragastric tube. For this purpose a very fine plastic tube (Clinifeed) is particularly useful and free from dangerous complications.

5 Level of Consciousness

Exact observations to measure the level of consciousness are difficult but the most generally used technique is the Glasgow Coma Scale described by Jennett and Teasdale.* There is no place for such terms as semicoma which have no real meaning. The coma scale observations are made and recorded 4-hourly by the nursing staff.

Three observations are made. These concern opening of the eyes, the response to a painful stimulus and the ability to speak. A score is given according to the response in each category:

Eye Opening	4	normal
	3	the eyes open in response to speech
	2	the eyes open in response to pain
	1	the eyes do not open at all
Speech	5	normal conversation
	4	confused
	3	some speech but not a conversation with another person.
	2	impossible to understand
	1	no speech at all
Motor response		Response to a painful stimulus such as strong pressure on the ridge of bone above the eye (the supraorbital ridge).
	5	obeys commands
	4	the hand localises the painful stimulus by moving up towards the site of pain
	3	flexion of the arm but not towards the site of pain
	2	the arm extends instead of flexing
	1	no response to a painful stimulus

Using the scale it is possible for the patient to score a range from 3 to 14. It is the progress which is made from hour to hour and from day to day which is important in the assessment of the patient's level of consciousness.

*For further study the student should read: *Management of Head Injuries* by Jennett, B., and Teasdale, G. (F. A. Davis Company, Philadelphia).

6   Nursing Care of Pressure Areas in an Unconscious Patient

Pressure necrosis of tissues is caused by continued compression of tissue between the bed and some boney point in the patient. In normal subjects there is constant natural movement even during sleep so that ischaemia caused by compression is relieved by movement and another part of the body is compressed. In this way no part of the body is compressed for a sufficient time for it to die as a result of compression which stops the flow of blood. Obviously this natural mechanism does not take place in a patient who is unconscious or paralysed and in these patients the natural process has to be replaced by action of the nursing staff.

The most common site for pressure necrosis is over the sacrum. With the patient lying on his back, the skin and fatty tissue is compressed between the sacrum and the bed. Another site is behind the heel, where the tissues are compressed against the heel bone (os calcis). If the patient is lying on the side, a common site for a pressure necrosis is the skin and fat covering the greater trochanter of the femur. When tissue is compressed in this way the blood cannot flow freely in the compressed tissue and as a result it dies. The early appearance is that the dead tissue forms a black and smelly slough and this eventually separates leaving an ulcer which goes down to bone. It is important to remember that when pressure necrosis occurs the full depth of tissue between the skin and the underlying bone is involved.

Patients who are unable to move naturally must be turned every two hours. The patient may be on his back for two hours and then spend the next two hours on one side. Patients who cannot be turned are lifted and the pressurised area rubbed to help to restore the circulation.

A sheepskin rug is sometimes used but these tend to get hard after washing. Another useful technique is the use of a ripple bed which constantly transfers the weight through the rippling action of the mattress. However, there is no substitute for good nursing and two hourly turning.

It is traditional for nurses to rub something into the so-called pressure points. There is not much data to support the value of this but if anything is to be rubbed into the pressure areas as a preventive it is likely that some greasey application would be best.

Secondary Brain Damage

This usually results from the development of a haematoma within the skull. A strong membrane lines the inside of the skull. This membrane is called the dura mater and a haematoma may occur between the dura and the skull when it is called an extradural haematoma. A haematoma may also occur on the brain side of the dura and this is called an intradural haematoma. Sometimes this haematoma is between the dura and the brain and is called a subdural haematoma but it is often associated with an intracerebral haematoma (Fig. 64).

Intracranial haematoma may follow quite minor injuries so that a patient who is not seriously ill may go into a life-threatening situation in a matter of hours after the accident.

The suspicion of intracranial haematoma is based on the deteriorating level of consciousness based on the observations made by the nurses. In a number of cases of diffuse brain damage the patient returns to a normal level of consciousness only to deteriorate into an unconscious state again as cerebral compression develops. This is called the lucid interval and is a characteristic but uncommon presentation. Other signs of raised intracranial pressure which are sometimes present include vomiting and severe headache. The eye signs which result from pressure on the oculomotor nerve should be studied at regular intervals when the level of consciousness is deteriorating. On the side of the lesion the pupil is dilated and does not react to light. A dilated pupil is a late and serious sign of cerebral compression and with modern techniques it should be possible to make the diagnosis and to decompress the brain before the appearance of pupillary signs.

When confronted with signs of compression the surgeon has to decompress the brain with the utmost urgency. Generally there are no focal clinical signs to guide the surgeon in regard to the site of the haematoma. The investigations which are performed are:

1 An **X-ray** of the skull. This may be helpful as a fracture of the temporal bone is often associated with an underlying haematoma. All cases of head injury have the skull X-rayed but this is as often for medico-legal as surgical reasons.

2 The routine study in many centres in the world is an **arteriogram**. Radio-opaque material is injected into the carotid artery and X-rays taken to display the intracranial branches. When a haematoma is present the arteries are usually displaced by the haematoma from their normal position. In more sophisticated centres the patient is investigated by **computerised tomography**. This is a perfectly safe study as it is non-invasive and because of the accurate and detailed information which it gives it has revolutionised the investigation of head injuries.

When a diagnosis of intracranial haematoma is made the treatment is by immediate operation. A flap of skull is raised to expose and evacuate the haematoma. The postoperative nursing care continues on the same lines as has already been described in dealing with a head injury.

Fracture of the Skull

There are several types of fracture of the skull which are diagnosed by X-ray.

1   *Fissured Fracture of the Vault*

Most fractures of the vault appear as long fissures. In itself this type of fracture has no significance except to indicate that a considerable injury has taken place. No treatment is directed to a fissured fracture.

2   *Fracture of the Base of the Skull*

This also indicates that a considerable trauma has been exerted on the skull and again no treatment is required for the fracture. However, a fracture of the base may cross the frontal or ethmoid sinuses of the nose and create a communication between the subarachnoid fluid surrounding the brain and the nose. The clinical manifestation of this is that blood and also cerebrospinal fluid drips from the nostril. The fracture may also cross the middle ear and result in the dripping of cerebrospinal fluid from the ear. These symptoms are called cerebrospinal otorrhea and cerebrospinal rhinorrhoea. The obvious risk is that infection may reach the subarachnoid space from the nose or ear and cause meningitis.

A cerebrospinal leak usually seals itself in a few days and reliance is put upon antibiotics to prevent meningitis. The nose or ear should not be plugged as this prevents free drainage and encourages infection.

3   *Depressed Fracture*

This type of localised fracture with depression of the fragments results from a localised injury. About half the cases follow road traffic accidents and one third occur at work. About 15 % result from assault.

Depressed fracture of the skull is important because the object which caused the fracture usually damages the skin so that the fracture is a compound one. As the dura is often injured too there is a risk of intracranial infection such as a localised abscess or meningitis. The brain damage is usually localised to the area of the depression so that unconsciousness is not usually present or is of short duration. Epilepsy is a late complication of depressed fracture if the depression is over the appropriate part of the brain. The risk of epilepsy is not significantly altered by elevating the fragments. In spite of this it is usual to operate on patients with a depressed fracture. The wound is cleaned and debrided under anaesthesia. The depressed fragments are elevated and the skin closed with sutures.

Chest Injuries

The most common chest injury is fracture of one or more ribs. This causes pain, particularly when the patient breathes deeply so that he tends to take shallow breaths and to use diaphragmatic movement to aerate the lungs. It is inadvisable to immobilise the chest with strapping as this further reduces the patient's ability to breathe and secretions are inclined to collect in the bronchi and cause lung collapse and infection. Opiates are also avoided as they depress respiration in addition to relieving pain. Fractured ribs always unite quickly and non-union is virtually unknown in spite of the fact that the rib ends are not immobilised. Pain can be relieved by giving an injection of local anaesthetic into the intercostal nerves which run from the back of the chest to the front in a little groove on the inner aspect of the rib which is called the intercostal groove.

An injection of long acting local anaesthetic (Marcaine) is made into two or three intercostal spaces at the level of the fracture.

Haemothorax and Pneumothorax

A rib fracture may be complicated by damage to the underlying lung which allows blood and air to collect in the pleural cavity. Air in the pleural cavity is called pneumothorax and a collection of blood in the pleural cavity is a haemothorax. In many cases there is a combination which is called haemopneumothorax. Proper lung function requires a clear airway and also a clear pleural cavity as the lung cannot expand if the pleural cavity is filled with air or blood. Patients with this complication may lose a lot of blood into the pleural cavity and go into hypovolaemic shock requiring blood transfusion. They may also be unable to get sufficient oxygen because of collapse of a lung.

Treatment of Haemopneumothorax (Fig. 65)

Once air and fluid are removed from the pleural cavity the lung expands to occupy the space. This is achieved by putting two tubes into the pleural cavity. Air rises to the top and a tube inserted into the second intercostal space in the front of the chest will release it. A second tube is put into the pleural space in the midaxillary line near the bottom of the chest cavity to drain blood. Blood drains easily from the pleural cavity because the constant movement caused by the heart beat and respiration interferes with the clotting mechanism and keeps it in liquid form.

The operation, which is an emergency, is done under local infiltration anaesthetic. The plastic tubes which are used have an inner

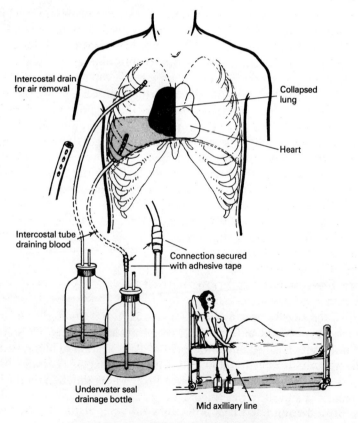

Intercostal drain for air removal

Collapsed lung

Heart

Intercostal tube draining blood

Connection secured with adhesive tape

Underwater seal drainage bottle

Mid axilliary line

This is the situation at the time of insertion of the drains
Air and blood are very quickly removed through the drains

Fig 65   Use of intercostal drains to drain air and blood from the pleural cavity

steel rod which is pointed to facilitate insertion (Argyll Co.). Once the tube is in the pleura the metal rod is removed and the plastic catheter attached to a tube which is connected to an underwater seal bottle containing a measured quantity of water. This is illustrated in Fig. 65. As the lung expands it displaces air and blood through the tube into the bottle. There are two tubes coming through the bung in each bottle. The long tube which is under the water is attached to the chest drain. Blood which drains is added to the water in the bottle and the amount can be measured. Air displaced from the tube is seen to bubble through the water seal and it then escapes from the second tube. When the lung is expanded the water in the bottle is seen to rise and fall in the tube with respiration. The pleural pressure is negative during inspiration when air is drawn into the lung and during this phase water rises in the tube. During expiration the water level falls.

The underwater drain allows the discharge of air and fluid from the chest but prevents the re-entry of air which would immediately fill the pleura and cause the lung to collapse. Although this device is very effective it is important that nurses should fully understand the principle as mismanagement of the tube and bottle can be disastrous.

1   All the tube connections should be taped together with zinc oxide plaster so that they cannot separate as a result of patient movement or ill-advised intervention of an assistant. If the tube is detached from the bottle the negative pressure inside the chest sucks air into the chest and causes a total pneumothorax and lung collapse.

If, for any reason, the tube needs to be disconnected, the Argyll tube is clamped with two pairs of strong artery forceps. It is then safe to detach the bottle for emptying and replacement without giving the patient a pneumothorax. The drain is reconnected to the bottle and secured with adhesive tape before the artery forceps are removed from the intercostal drain. Two forceps are always used in case one snaps off accidentally.

2   If the drain is connected to the wrong tube on the bottle the patient will get a total pneumothorax as soon as the clamp is removed.

3   If the bottle is lifted above the level of the chest the fluid will run into the chest and as the water seal is now gone the patient will get a pneumothorax. If there is any reason for lifting the bottle, such as during transportation of the patient from the theatre to the ward, the tube must be clamped with strong artery forceps before lifting the bottle.

4   Another mishap which sometimes occurs with the Argyll tube is that, if it has not been properly secured, it may slip partly out of the chest. The Argyll tube has a number of side openings to help with drainage and if some of these are inside the chest and some are outside

it is obvious that a pneuthorax will develop. The emergency treatment is to try to close the holes outside the chest by applying a vaseline gauze pack. Surgical help is requested urgently to replace the tube.

The postoperative care of a patient with a chest drain consists of encouraging deep breathing to aerate the lungs fully. A chest X-ray is taken daily and when the lung is fully expanded the tubes are removed from the chest.

Removal of an Intercostal Chest Drain

The risk involved in removing a chest drain is that air will enter the chest through the opening left by removal of the tube. There is inevitably a brief moment when some of the holes in the tube are within and some outside the chest so that the removal must be rapid to minimise the entry of air. The technique for removal of the tube is:

    1   The patient is told to take a deep breath and to hold it to expand the lung fully.

    2   The tube is rapidly removed from the chest. A useful technique to stop air entering the chest as the tube is removed is to place a square of carbonet round the tube at the skin opening to cover the hole as the tube is removed.

    3   Surgeons leave an untied suture in this wound and when the drain is removed a second nurse or doctor ties the suture under the carbonet to close the wound. The whole is then covered with an Elastoplast dressing.

There is always a possibility that air will enter the chest when a drain is removed and an X-ray of the chest is taken as soon as possible afterwards.

Abdominal Injuries

The abdominal contents may be damaged by penetrating injuries such as by a gunshot wound or knife or by violent external trauma which may particularly damage the liver, spleen or kidneys. Penetrating wounds are also likely to cut holes in the intestine so allowing the contents to escape and cause peritonitis.

The abdomen is a large cavity and contains very vascular organs whose injury results in haemorrhage into the peritoneum. Such bleeding can be very severe and cause hypovolaemic shock.

As with all accident surgery the treatment of hypovolaemic shock is instituted at once and if the surgeon decides that the blood loss is due to damage to some abdominal organ an early operation will be done.

Preoperative Studies

As an early operation is likely to be required, the patient must not be allowed anything by mouth. Collection of a urine sample is important as blood in the urine is a constant sign of injury to the urinary tract. In the abscence of any sign of injury to the pelvis haematuria is nearly always due to kidney trauma.

A plain X-ray of the abdomen is often taken but is not generally very useful.

If the surgeon is in doubt he may insert a needle into the peritoneal cavity in each of the four quadrants. If blood is aspirated it is certain that some organ in the abdomen has been damaged.

Rupture of the Spleen

The spleen is often damaged in major accidents but, especially in children, it may rupture as a result of a comparatively minor fall. The spleen is located under the left dome of the diaphragm and pain is felt in the upper left abdomen and also in the left shoulder. This pain is very typical of splenic rupture and is an example of referred pain. The nerves to the shoulder and also to the diaphragm come from the same cervical segments (mainly cervical 4), so that pain can be felt in the shoulder although the lesion is in the diaphragm or pressing on it.

If the spleen is found to be damaged and the patient is more than ten years old it is best and safest to remove it (splenectomy). The spleen is the source of many of the cells which are responsible for immunity to infections and it is surprising that the operation of splenectomy does not cause serious impairment of the immune response when it is performed in adults. However, there is evidence that in children and particularly in infants, splenectomy may be followed by impaired immunity to infection which may be serious. For this reason the surgeon tries to conserve the spleen when dealing with young children and to pack the wound with absorbable haemostatic gauze.

The postoperative management does not usually call for any special measures apart from the routine observations. However, when the spleen has not been removed there is a risk of recurrent haemorrhage and it is necessary to pay special attention to the postoperative observations such as pulse rate and blood pressure so that signs of recurrent haemorrhage will be detected.

Fractures

One or more fractures may complicate any major accident with multiple injuries or a fracture may be an isolated injury.

There are four principles in the treatment of fractures:

   1   The bones are manipulated into a position as near to normal as is possible. This is called reduction.

   2   Following reduction some technique is used to fix the bones in position so maintaining the reduction.

   3   Immobilisation of the bones is maintained until union has taken place.

   4   During the period of immobilisation attention is directed to maintaining function in the muscles and joints of the limb. This part of the treatment is undertaken and supervised by members of the physiotherapy department.

Types of Fracture

   1   The break may be transverse or spiral. Once a transverse facture has been reduced it is relatively easy to maintain but an oblique or spiral fracture tends to slip and requires more secure fixation (Fig. 66).

   2   A comminuted fracture is one in which there is splintering or fragmentation of the bone ends.

   3   A complicated fracture is one associated with an injury to some other important structure such as a main artery or nerve (Fig. 69).

   4   A compound fracture is one which is associated with an overlying skin injury. This may be caused by the agent causing the

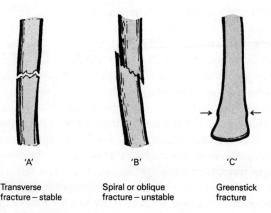

'A'   'B'   'C'

Transverse   Spiral or oblique   Greenstick
fracture – stable   fracture – unstable   fracture

Fig 66 Types of fracture

trauma or the broken bone ends may have penetrated the skin. The danger of a compound fracture is the possibility of infection of the bone and an important part of the treatment of a compound fracture is to convert it to a simple fracture by closure of the skin as soon as possible.

5   A fracture is said to be impacted when the broken ends are fixed together.

6   In children the bones are more elastic and less brittle and sometimes the bone breaks on only one side resulting in some bending or no deformity at all. This is called a greenstick fracture (Fig. 66).

Spontaneous Fractures

Considerable force is required to break a normal bone. When a fracture takes place with minimal trauma or with no trauma at all, the fracture is called spontaneous or pathological.

The most common cause of a spontaneous fracture is osteoporosis, which is an affection of the elderly in which the amount of actual bone tissue in the bones is diminished so weakening the structure. This is called idiopathic osteoporosis because the cause is unknown and there is no effective treatment. Osteoporosis also occurs as a result of disuse and may be seen in bones which have been immobilised for a long time. Patients on long term steroid therapy also develop osteoporosis.

Primary or secondary bone tumours may result in spontaneous fracture and secondary deposits of breast cancer causing fracture of the neck or shaft of the femur is a common surgical problem.

Early Management of Fractures

1   *Immobilisation in a plaster cast*

The classical technique for the immobilisation of a fracture is to encase the part in a close fitting plaster cast which usually immobilises the joints above and below the fracture. This type of immobilisation is used in some fractures of the leg and ankle and in wrist fractures.

Colles' Fracture.   Colles' fracture is a spontaneous fracture occurring in elderly people as a result of a fall on the outstretched hand. In a normal young person no fracture would result but in an older person with idiopathic osteoporosis the radius fractures about 2 cm above the wrist joint. The lower fragment is displaced backwards and impacts into the upper part of the radius giving rise to a typical appearance which is called the 'Dinner Fork' deformity.

Colles' fracture requires reduction under a local or short general anaesthetic. After reduction the part is immobilised in a Plaster of Paris cast which extends from the knuckles to just below the elbow joint.

All plaster casts in whatever part of the body are subject to one very serious and dangerous complication. If swelling takes place at the fracture site the part cannot expand externally because of the unyielding cast and the underlying limb is compressed. If this condition is unrecognised and untreated the compression becomes so severe that the blood flow is arrested as if a tourniquet had been applied and the limb becomes gangrenous beyond the point of compression. It is most important to observe patients very carefully during the first 6– 12 hours after the application of a cast. If the plaster becomes too tight because of swelling the patient will complain of severe pain under the cast. The hand beyond the cast swells because the compression obstructs the return of blood in the veins and as the compression becomes more severe the patient is unable to move the fingers and the hand becomes anaesthetised. These effects are caused by the reduction of arterial blood supply to the nerves which cease to function.

If the nurse is concerned that the plaster has become too tight she should seek medical assistance immediately. The only effective and safe remedy is to split the cast from end to end to release the pressure and restore the flow of blood. Elevation may help to reduce swelling but if there are signs of circulatory obstruction the cast must be split.

2   Treatment by Internal Fixation

Many fractures are now immobilised with metal plates, screws, etc. In the early days of this work the introduction of large foreign bodies was often followed by infection and the screws and other metal materials loosened very quickly because of corrosion. Infection is now much less common and the metal used is stainless steel which is completely inert.

Fractures of the long bones, especially the shaft of the femur, can be treated by an operation in which a long rod is passed through the medullary cavity of the bone extending well above and below the fracture. This is called a Kuntscher intramedullary nail. Young patients with this type of fracture used to be kept in bed many weeks but they are now able to put weight on the leg and to walk on the day following the introduction of a Kuntscher nail (Fig. 69).

3 Fractures of the Neck of the Femur

At the upper end of the femur there are two large lumps of bone which are called the greater and lesser trochanters. These are for the attachment of muscles and give a better mechanical advantage. Above this point the neck of the femur slopes at an angle and is surmounted by the rounded head which fits into the acetabulum of the pelvis making the hip joint (Fig. 67).

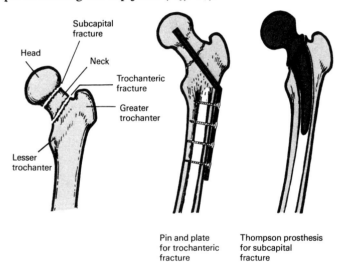

Subcapital fracture

Head

Neck

Trochanteric fracture

Greater trochanter

Lesser trochanter

Pin and plate for trochanteric fracture

Thompson prosthesis for subcapital fracture

Fig 67 Fracture of the neck of the femur

Fractures of the neck of the femur are common in elderly women and, like the Colles' fracture, they are spontaneous caused by idiopathic osteoporosis and resulting from very minor falls. Such a fracture is impossible to immobilise with an external cast and before the days of internal fixation it was a virtual death sentence. The elderly patient was in pain and unable to walk. Confined to bed early death from pneumonia was usual. These fractures are now treated surgically. If the fracture is at the level of the trochanters (trochanteric fracture) a nail can be passed through the fracture and to give this secure fixation it is attached to a steel plate which is screwed to the shaft of the femur. There are several types but a Jewett nail and plate is often used.

When the fracture is below the head (subcapital) it is impossible to immobilise safely as the head is too small for a secure hold. These cases are treated by excision of the head and neck of the femur and the whole is replaced by a steel head and neck called a Thompson prosthesis (Fig. 67).

This formation of a new hip joint is called an arthroplasty.

Postoperative Care. Following surgical treatment of a fractured neck of the femur the patient is able to take some weight and to walk on the day following the operation. The physiotherapist is asked to assist with breathing and mobilisation of the patient and with exercises to maintain full function of the limb.

Arterial Injuries

In England today the most common cause of an arterial injury is a road traffic accident. The injury usually results from a severe degree of violence and is often associated with a fracture and serious injuries in other parts of the body. In more violent societies, knife and gunshot wounds account for a high percentage of injuries and knife wounds are now becoming more common in this country. At the same time, with increasing attention to safety at work, factory accidents are less common and usually occur when safety regulations have been disregarded.

Types of Injury

1   **Complete Division of the Artery.**   This is most commonly associated with a knife injury and may be accompanied by severe bleeding. When the artery is completely divided the two ends retract and contract reducing the blood loss.

2   **Partial division** is also frequently caused by penetrating injury. Bleeding from the injured artery is often very considerable. When the artery is deeply placed, the blood lost is confined in the body by fascial planes and forms a large haematoma. The peripheral part of this haematoma clots in layers but the part of the haematoma near to the artery remains as liquid blood. This is called a false aneurysm or

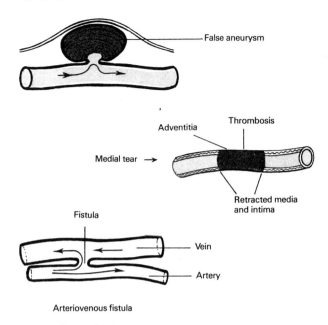

False aneurysm

Adventitia

Thrombosis

Medial tear →

Retracted media
and intima

Fistula

Vein

Artery

Arteriovenous fistula

Fig 68 Types of arterial injury

pulsating haematoma (Fig. 68). The outstanding clinical feature of a false aneurysm is the expansile pulsation of the lump and the loud murmur which can be heard with the stethoscope. A false aneurysm sometimes grows in size and may also throw off fragments of blood clot (emboli) which will block more peripheral arteries causing acute ischaemia which may threaten survival of the limb. False aneurysms are usually treated surgically.

3 Arteriovenous Fistula. If the penetrating injury damages the artery and its accompanying vein at the same time, the blood escaping from the artery may flow into the low pressure vein forming a communication which is called an arteriovenous fistula. The flow of blood through a fistula causes dramatic symptoms. There is a palpable thrill like the purring of a cat over the site of the fistula and this sound is easily heard with a stethoscope and is sometimes loud enough to be heard by the patient. The blood passing through the fistula returns immediately to the heart so that in addition to the normal amount of blood pumped by the heart there is also the recirculation of blood which has been through the fistula. This increase in cardiac output may eventually cause cardiac failure.

An arteriovenous fistula is treated by division of the fistula and reconstruction of the artery and vein.

4 **Medial Tear.**   There are three layers in the wall of an artery:
   (a)   The outer layer is called the adventitia.
   (b)   The inner layer, which is called the intima, consists of flattened cells which have the unique property of allowing blood to pass without causing coagulation.
   (c)   The media is the main part of the artery wall and consists of muscle and elastic tissue. Contraction of the muscle reduces the lumen of the artery and lessens the flow of blood. During hypovolaemic shock the muscles in the arteries all over the body contract to reduce the flow and this contributes to preventing further fall in the blood pressure. When an artery is injured the muscle contracts so reducing the blood loss. Muscle contraction (or spasm) also occurs in the arteries of a limb which has been injured even when the main artery is intact. Spasm sometimes gives rise to effects similar to those seen when an artery is injured and the distinction may be difficult. The other component of the media is the elastic fibres. Every time the heart contracts blood is pumped into the arteries which expand and this is the pulse which you feel at the wrist. Following a heart beat the elastic fibres in the artery cause an elastic recoil which causes the artery to return to its former diameter.

When an artery is subjected to a severe blunt injury and at the same time stretched, the intima and media are likely to rupture round the circumference of the artery. The loose adventitia layer remains intact so that when the artery is seen at an operation it looks externally almost normal. However, when the media is divided it retracts because of its elastic properties. This leaves about 2 cm of artery which is not lined with intima and in this short length of artery the blood comes into contact with the adventitia and very soon thromboses causing acute ischaemia (Fig. 68). This injury is commonly associated with a major fracture such as the lower third of the femur, where the main artery is in contact with the femur.

A patient with a medial tear and a short segment of thrombosis in a main artery will come into hospital with the signs of acute ischaemia. The limb will seem cool when compared with the normal side and the colour will change to very pale or later to blotchy patches of blue. The important signs that the limb is not viable are that the patient is unable to move the toes and the limb becomes anaesthetic. These signs are due to the fact that the nerves cease to function when the blood supply is dangerously low.

The treatment of acute ischaemia due to a medial tear is immediate operation. The fracture is immobilised, usually with an intramedullary nail, and the thrombosed segment of artery excised and replaced with a graft of saphenous vein (Fig. 69).

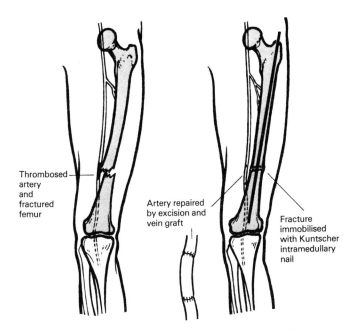

Thrombosed artery and fractured femur

Artery repaired by excision and vein graft

Fracture immobilised with Kuntscher intramedullary nail

Fig 69 Fracture of shaft of femur complicated by medial tear and thrombosis of femoral artery

Postoperative Management

The usual postoperative observations are made but there are special considerations in cases of artery repair.

1 Haemorrhage.   Traumatic cases are not usually heparinised because of the risk of bleeding from the damaged tissue. A suction drain is placed in the wound but haemorrhage from the suture line is usually retained in the tissues and a haematoma develops. The operation site is inspected at intervals and if a haematoma develops the doctor is informed. Occasionally it will be necessary to return the patient to the operating room to stop the bleeding.

2   In some cases the acute ischaemia recurs, possibly because of thrombosis at the site of the artery repair. It is important to nurse the patient with the feet exposed so that any colour change can be seen easily and without too much disturbance of the patient. Other signs of recurrent ischaemia will be coolness of the skin and loss of skin sensation. In healthy young adults return of the foot pulses is likely after repair of an artery and the site of the pulse on the foot is usually marked with ink. The pulse should be observed at 15 minute intervals and disappearance reported to the doctor, although loss of the pulse does not necessarily mean that the main artery has rethrombosed.

Management of burns

A major burn usually causes great pain and anxiety. The patient needs mental support and reassurance, especially in the early stages.

The problems of management depend on many factors but the depth of the burn is one of the most important. The skin comprises two layers. The superficial layer is called the epidermis and consists of a basal layer from which the more superficial cells are derived by division. As cells are produced from the basal layer the cells at the surface are shed. If a limb remains bandaged for some weeks a shower of white flakes appears when the bandage is removed. These are the superficial cells which have been desquamated. Underneath the epidermis is an elastic layer called the dermis which contains the hair roots and the sweat glands.

There are a number of different ways in which burns are classified but a simple classification is into partial skin loss (superficial) and the whole skin loss (deep). If the burn is superficial to the basal layer, skin can regenerate from it and spontaneous healing will result. But if the burn is deep and destroys the basal layer there is no possibility of regeneration of normal skin and the burned area can never heal.

The treatment of burns is specialised and the results are greatly improved if patients are treated in a Burns Unit under the care of a Plastic Surgery Unit.

Primary Treatment

During the first 36 to 48 hours there is a great deal of protein rich exudate from the burned area. This fluid loss results in hypovolaemic shock because the fluid is drawn from the tissue spaces and from the circulating blood. If the blood pressure is allowed to remain low the patient will develop acute renal failure. The emergency treatment during this time is the replacement of sufficient fluid to keep the blood pressure and renal output normal. In some units an electrolyte solution such as Hartmann's solution is used for fluid replacement but a solution containing protein is a more satisfactory replacement and Human Purified Protein Fraction (HPPF) is given in some centres.

In a severe burn, a urinary catheter is used to measure the urine output and the aim should be to keep it at about 50 ml an hour. Regular measurements of the pulse rate and blood pressure are also used to assess the state of shock. Patients with severe burns develop a severe anaemia and many units of blood may be required to restore the haemoglobin to normal.

Pain is likely to be severe in the early stages and relief with morphine or other drugs will be required.

Local Treatment

There has been some debate concerning the best local treatment. For some years the burn was left exposed to heal if it was superficial or to form an eschar of dead tissue if it was deep. Recently there has been a return to the idea that the burn is best kept moist as this seems to save more skin.

Infection is one of the great problems of burns as it causes the death of skin which was just viable and makes grafting impossible. All dressings are done with the strictest aseptic technique and carriers are not allowed to work in the unit until cleared of infection. Antibiotics are not used because of the risk of infection with bacteria such as *Pseudomonas pyocyanea* which are resistant to most antibiotics. However, an antibacterial dressing controls infection and 1% Flamazine cream, which is silver sulphadiazine, is smeared onto the whole of the burn and this is covered with layers of gauze to absorb the fluid exudate. If the exudate comes through the gauze dressings a plastic sheet may be used to contain it. In the case of hand burns, the hand is covered in Flamazine cream and placed in a sterile plastic bag where free movement of the fingers is possible unencumbered by dressings.

At the end of about two weeks a partial skin burn is healed but a total skin burn shows an area of burned skin which is now a grey slough beginning to separate from the underlying tissue. At this stage the patient is taken to the operating theatre and the dead skin removed under a general anaesthetic. Split skin grafts are used to cover defects. If the burn is very extensive it is possible to get temporary cover with cadaver skin or even with pig skin, but although these foreign grafts take they are quickly rejected and they are no substitute for the patients own skin.

Nutrition

Although much of the protein lost in the exudate is replaced by transfusion, patients with severe burns lose weight and need extra nutrition. If the patient cannot be tempted to eat enough, the diet has to be supplemented with intragastric feeding using a fine plastic tube in the stomach or in some cases by intravenous feeding.

Trauma Involving the Urinary Tract

Renal Injury

The kidney can be injured by a penetrating injury such as a knife or gunshot wound, or by blunt external trauma. In either case the injury may be isolated or there may be coincidental injury of adjacent structures. These include damage to the spleen, fracture of the lower ribs, and possibly intrathoracic injuries.

The injury may be unnoticed when it is an accidental kick during a game of rugby football but kicks in the loin of a victim involved in a vicious attack are often responsible for renal injury. There may be a minor tear in the cortex or a more extensive tear into a calyx. In the worst cases the kidney is shattered.

The outstanding symptom of renal injury is haematuria but some loin pain is usual. There may be considerable bleeding around the kidney and this is sometimes sufficient to cause hypovolaemic shock.

Management of a Patient with a Renal Injury

As with all cases of trauma, the first consideration is to make the usual observations of blood pressure and pulse rate and to replace blood if there are signs of shock.

Most cases of renal injury stop bleeding within 48 hours and it is essential to save all specimens of urine which are passed to assess the amount of bleeding. So long as the bleeding is getting less a conservative regime is pursued.

An intravenous urogram is done at an early stage to see that there is a normal kidney on the opposite side. In serious cases in which the bleeding does not stop and blood transfusion continues to be needed the surgeon will have to explore the kidney to stop the bleeding. In most cases this operation will end up with removal of the kidney, but it is essential to have a urogram before the operation to ensure that the second kidney is present and of reasonable function before doing a nephrectomy. Patients with renal trauma are generally kept in the hospital for at least ten days because although the bleeding usually stops within 48 hours there is a risk of severe secondary haemorrhage. This will present with recurrent haematuria and will be treated with bedrest and blood transfusion if hypovolaemic shock is present. Like primary haemorrhage it is likely that a secondary haemorrhage will stop spontaneously within 48 hours.

Injuries to the Male Urethra

The anatomy of the male urethra is illustrated in Fig. 70. The urethra may be damaged in two places:

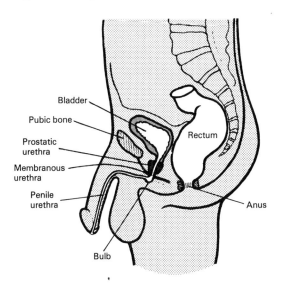

Fig 70 The male urethra

I The Perineal Urethra or Bulb. The bulb of the urethra is the widest part and is situated in the perineum below the external sphincter of the bladder. Classically it is described as being caused by falling astride. However, it more often results from being attacked by kicking while the victim is lying on the ground. The urethra is severely injured and bruised so that there is no possibility of immediate suture.

When the bulb of the urethra is damaged there will be blood dribbling from the urethra and pain and swelling in the perineum. If the patient tries to pass urine some will pass out of the hole into the tissues. This is called extravasation of urine and the urine seeps through the tissues passing forwards across the scrotum and then up the anterior abdominal wall. Infection of this tissue containing extravasated urine results in gangrene of all the subcutaneous tissue covering the perineum, scrotum and lower anterior abdominal wall. To avoid this catastrophe it is essential to implore the patient not to try to pass urine if a rupture of the bulb is suspected.

The immediate treatment is a suprapubic cystotomy to divert the urine and so prevent extravasation. The urethra heals spontaneously but although some patients may have no further trouble a notorious complication is the formation of a stricture of the urethra. This means that during the healing process too much fibrosis takes place resulting in narrowing of the urethra by the scar.

2   Rupture of the Membranous Urethra.   This injury is always caused by a fracture of the pelvis. The prostate gland lies immediately behind the pubic bone which is a part of the pelvis. If the pubic bone is displaced backwards as a result of the fracture it carries the bladder and prostate back and this shears off the urethra below the prostate. This part of the urethra is called the membranous urethra.

When there is a fracture of the pelvis with displacement of the pubis there is a possibility of rupture of the urethra. The clinical signs are dribbling of blood from the urethra and inability to pass urine.

In some cases the lesion is partial but in others there is wide separation of the two ends of the urethra.

A number of different techniques are in use for these cases but most are treated by suprapubic cystotomy. In some cases the surgeon is able to pass a catheter through the urethra and another through the urethral opening in the bladder. If these two can be made to meet the urethral catheter can be steered into the bladder across the rupture and left in position while the urethra heals. Many patients with a rupture of the membranous urethra end up with a stricture.

23

Tracheostomy

Tracheostomy is an operation in which a curved tube is placed in an opening which the surgeon makes in the trachea just below the larynx. This serious operation may be temporary or permanent. The indications are:

1   Inadequate respiration caused by fractured ribs (flail chest) or more often by depressed respiratory function. This situation often follows major operations or major trauma. In the first instance the patient is treated by endotracheal intubation (Fig. 63) but this cannot be used indefinitely and if respiratory support is still required after a period which varies from 7 to 21 days the endotracheal tube will be replaced by a tracheostomy. Some tracheostomy tubes are fitted with a balloon which can be inflated to completely occlude the trachea. This prevents the escape of air or oxygen which is used under pressure from a respirator to inflate the lungs. Some doctors advise regular deflation of the balloon to prevent pressure necrosis of the lining of the trachea but this is not universal practice.

2   An emergency tracheostomy may also be required if there is obstruction to the airway in the pharynx or larynx. This may be the result of inflammation, oedema which may follow the sting of a wasp, or paralysis of the vocal cords.

3   Permanent tracheostomy may be necessary following removal of the larynx (laryngectomy). This operation is done in some cases of cancer of the larynx.

Management of Tracheostomy

1   For emergency tracheostomy, a tube made of soft plastic is used. The tube is secured in position with tapes which encircle the neck and a small foam dressing is placed between the wound and the tracheostomy tube. Displacement of the tracheostomy tube can be a disaster as an acute respiratory emergency results and the doctor must be called at once. Replacement of a tracheostomy tube may be very difficult and in an emergency it may be easier to restore the airway by passing an endotracheal tube through the mouth.

2   Drying and encrustation of the lining of the trachea results from the inspiration of air which has not been humidified by passing

through the nose on the way to the trachea. To overcome this problem the patient is given air or oxygen which is humidified by passage through a humidifier. Drying can also be prevented by the use of a spray of normal saline and the injection of 3 to 5 ml of normal saline into the tracheostomy immediately before aspiration.

3   Infection and the collection of tracheal and bronchial secretions causes obstruction to the passage of gases through the trachea. Regular aspiration of the trachea and bronchi is done by passing a sterile catheter through the tracheostomy. This must be done as a sterile procedure using gloves and a sterile, disposable catheter connected to a suction line. During aspiration there is often a dramatic fall in the level of oxygen in the blood and a second nurse is required to administer oxygen at every opportunity during the aspiration.

The maintenance of a clear airway is an essential part of tracheostomy management and the equipment needed for aspiration must be kept on the bedside locker as tracheal obstruction requires immediate relief. A conscious patient is given a bell to call for assistance if he feels that his respiration is obstructed. The introduction of infection directly into the air passages as a result of faulty technique is a disaster.

Physiotherapy is an essential part of the care of a patient with a tracheostomy. It assists the flow of secretions from the lung and bronchi into the main bronchi and trachea where they can be removed by aspiration.

A tracheostomy tube is removed when respiratory function is restored to normal. A small dressing is placed over the opening which may be expected to close very quickly.

Permanent Tracheostomy

This operation is usually done following removal of the larynx for cancer. The early management is the same as for a temporary tracheostomy but before going home the patient is fitted with a Negus type silver tracheostomy tube. This tube has an separate inner tube which can be removed without displacement of the outer tracheostomy tube. The inner tube can then be cleaned with chlorhexidine in spirit (Hibitane) and replaced.

24

The Urinary Tract

Urine is manufactured from blood in the kidneys which are situated at the back of the abdomen just below the diaphragm. The urine is collected into a pouch of the kidney called the pelvis. It then passes down a tube about 25 cm long (the ureter) to enter the bladder which is a muscular reservoir in which the urine is collected and stored. The bladder can be emptied by the patient at will. This is called micturition.

Anatomy and Physiology of the Kidney (Fig. 71)

On looking at the cut surface of a kidney it can be seen that there is an outer rim about 6—7 mm wide which is called the cortex and an inner

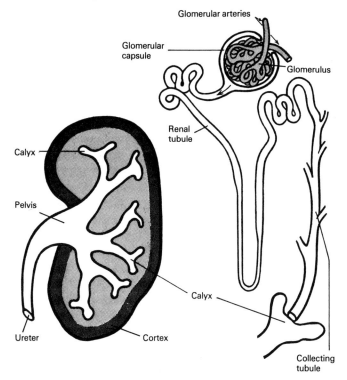

Fig 71   Anatomy and microanatomy of the kidney

part which is the medulla. The initial process of manufacture of urine is one of filtration in the renal corpuscle (glomerular corpuscle). Each renal corpuscle is about 0.2 mm in diameter and there are about one million in each kidney. A tiny tuft of capillary blood vessels invaginate the end of each renal tubule as one might push in the end of the finger of a glove. This forms a little capsule around the capillary tuft which is called the glomerular capsule (Bowman's capsule) into which urine is filtered from the blood (glomerular filtration). The huge scale of this operation working with more than two million renal corpuscles results in the filtration of about 170 litres of urine every 24 hours. As the fluid passes from the glomerular capsule into the renal tubules the composition and quantity of this fluid is greatly modified. A great deal of the water is reabsorbed back into the blood so conserving fluid and preventing dehydration. Sodium, chloride, glucose, amino acids and other substances are also reabsorbed. The reabsorption of water is controlled by a hormone secreted by the pituitary gland and called the antidiuretic hormone. Following removal or disease of the pituitary gland the patient may not be able to absorb water in the renal tubules and will pass a huge amount of urine. This disease is called diabetes insipidus.

The urine is therefore produced in gross form in the glomerular capsule and then modified in the renal tubules. These two parts of the kidney are collectively called the nephrone.

Once the urine is formed it is collected in tubes called the collecting tubules which join together and finally discharge into a collecting space called a calyx. Several calyces join to form the pelvis of the kidney which is continuous with the ureter.

Anatomy and Physiology of the Bladder (Fig. 72)

The bladder occupies a position in the pelvis immediately behind the pubic bone. In the male the rectum is behind the bladder but in the female the uterus and vagina are interposed between the bladder and the rectum. The bladder acts as a reservoir of urine which is constantly received from the kidneys via the ureters. As urine fills the bladder the muscle of the bladder which is called the detrusor muscle lengthens to enlarge the reservoir without any rise in the intravesical pressure. When about 150 to 200 ml of urine are in the bladder the muscle is so stretched that a nervous impulse is sent to the spinal cord. A return signal from the spinal cord which is called a spinal reflex causes a contraction of the bladder. In infancy and in patients with an injury to the spinal cord this return signal causes immediate emptying of the

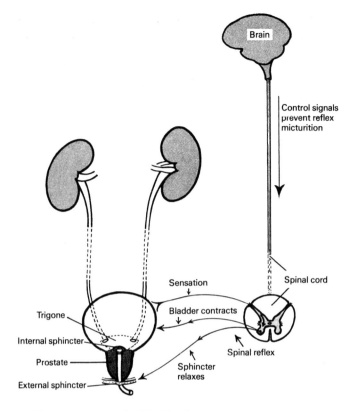

Fig 72 The nervous control of bladder function

bladder. However, in normal adults the spinal reflex is controlled by nerve signals from the brain and after a mild contraction of the bladder which is felt as a desire to pass urine the return signal is stopped and micturition does not take place. In normal adults the bladder emptying reflex can be initiated at will by nerve signals which come from the brain to instruct the spinal reflex to operate and cause bladder contraction. The spinal reflex concerned with bladder emptying is at the level of the second and third sacral nerve segments.

Operations on the rectum and uterus may damage the nerves of this reflex and this results in varying degrees of interference with bladder emptying.

The reflex operates without inhibition from the brain if there is a lesion of the spinal cord above the level of the reflex which prevents the passage of nerve signals from the brain to the level of the spinal reflex. Such lesions may be an injury of the cord following fracture dislocation of the spine or certain neurological lesions such as multiple sclerosis which may occur in the spinal cord.

There are two sphincters at the bladder outlet. The internal sphincter is at the neck of the bladder and cannot have any effect on urinary continence as it is destroyed in the operation of prostatectomy without inducing incontinence. The internal sphincter is part of the male sexual mechanism and closes during ejaculation to prevent reflux ejaculation into the bladder. Following prostatectomy reflux ejaculation is usual. The external sphincter is below the prostate and relaxes when the detrusor muscle contracts.

Anatomy and Physiology of the Male Genital System (Fig. 73)

The anatomy and function of the male generative organs are closely related to the urinary system.

Testicle

The testicle is made up of two parts which are called the testis and the epididymis. The testis is the organ in which the male germ cells called spermatozoa are made. It is also the site of production of the male hormone testosterone. During development of the embryo the testes

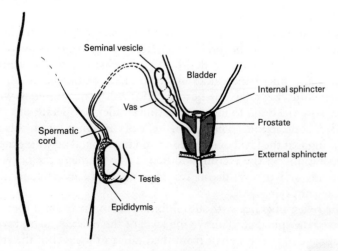

Fig 73   The anatomy of the male genital system

develop at the back of the abdomen and migrate to their normal position in the scrotum just before birth. Failure of this normal descent to take place results in the condition of undescended testicle in which the testicle is usually found somewhere in the anterior abdominal wall and rarely inside the abdominal cavity. The epididymis is attached to the back of the testis. It is a long convoluted tube through which the spermatozoa have to pass on leaving the testis. Abnormal spermatozoa are destroyed and absorbed in the epididymis. The testicle is encased by a sac called the tunica vaginalis which contains a small amount of fluid and affords some protection against injury.

Seminal Vesicles and Prostate

After passing through the epididymis the spermatozoa find themselves in a straight tube called the vas deferens. The vas runs with the vessels of the spermatic cord and is easily found by surgeons because its very thick wall and small lumen make it easy to identify. This fact is made use of in the operation of vasectomy in which the vas is picked up and divided through a very small incision.

The vas passes through the prostate gland and opens into the prostatic urethra. Just before it enters the prostate it is joined by a pouch which lies behind the bladder and which is called the seminal vesicle. The seminal vesicle secretes and holds about 5 ml of seminal fluid. Spermatozoa are stored in the terminal part of the vas. The prostate is a muscular and glandular organ situated below the bladder. It is pierced by the prostatic urethra.

The Penis

The penis consists of three cylindrical parts which are encased in a thick unyielding layer called Buck's fascia. One cylinder called the corpus spongiosum is traversed by the penile urethra. The other two are paired and are called the corpora cavernosa. All three corpora have a rich arterial supply but in the flaccid state the blood passes through shunts directly into the veins which carry blood away from the penis. During erection the shunts are closed and blood is retained in the large vascular spaces of the corpora which become rigid because of their encasement in the unyielding layer of fascia.

The expanded end of the corpus spongiosum through which the urethra opens is called the glans penis and is covered by a retractile hood of skin (prepuce or foreskin).

Ejaculation

Contraction of the seminal vesicles causes ejaculation of the seminal fluid which picks up and shunts out the sperm rich fluid contained in the terminal part of the vas. Contractions of the prostate gland probably contribute to the ejaculation of fluid but only a minute volume of semen comes from the prostate, the main bulk coming from the seminal vesicles. Closure of the internal bladder sphincter prevents the semen from entering the bladder.

Semen normally contains about 50 million spermatozoa in each ml of fluid and a normal ejaculation is about 5 ml.

Investigation of a Urological Patient

Urine Testing

This task, which usually falls to the nursing staff, has been greatly simplified by the introduction of sensitised papers which change colour if the urine contains a particular abnormal constituent such as sugar, albumin, blood or bile. Reference to a colour scale gives a quantitative result.

Infection in the urinary tract is common and specimens of urine are sent for bacteriological examination. Bacteria are normally present on the urethral meatus and the adjacent urethra. After cleansing the meatus the patient is instructed to pass urine allowing the first part of the specimen to go to waste and collecting the rest in a sterile urine specimen container. In this way the urethral organisms do not contaminate the specimen.

Blood Tests

The blood urea is derived from the break down of exogenous protein (i.e. protein taken in as food) as well as endogenous protein (i.e. body protein). It is a routine test of renal function in many laboratories and the level is raised if there is impairment of renal function. In patients who are dehydrated because of some acute surgical emergency such as intestinal obstruction the level is also raised because there is insufficient excretion of water.

The blood creatinine is solely derived from endogenous protein and is a more reliable indicator of urinary function than the blood urea. The test is a creatinine clearance test which estimates the rate of clearance of creatinine from the blood.

X-ray Examination

1 A plain film of the abdomen should show the outline of the kidneys and bladder. Opaque urinary stones are also shown.

2 **Excretion Urography.** In this test an intravenous dose of radio-opaque medium containing iodine is given to the patient. The only preparation is that the patient is fasted for 6 hours prior to the examination. At the completion of the injection the medium is already in the renal tubules. An X-ray taken at this time shows the medium in the solid part of the kidney and this is called a nephrogram. Within 2—3 minutes the medium has passed from the renal tubules to reach the calyces and pelvis of the kidney and later films show this part of the kidney. During this part of the examination strong compression is applied to the lower abdomen to compress the ureters so holding the medium in the kidney and enhancing the pictures. Later films show the ureters and bladder. A second film of the bladder after asking the patient to pass water gives a rough estimate of any residual urine which might be present as a result of bladder outflow obstruction.

Some patients are sensitive to iodine or some other constituent of the contrast medium and nausea and vomiting are common complications. Very severe reactions occur but are very rare. Minor reactions are probably exacerbated by anxiety and the patient should be encouraged as much as possible.

Renal Arteriogram

A catheter passed into the femoral artery at the groin can be manipulated so that the tip enters the renal artery. An injection of radio-opaque material given directly into the renal artery shows the renal circulation. This technique can be used to diagnose the nature of a lump found in the kidney. A cyst has no circulation but a carcinoma has a tumour circulation.

Needle Aspiration

This test is carried out in the X-ray department where the needle can be safely negotiated into the kidney lump under X-ray control. If a cyst is entered the typical fluid is aspirated. If the needle enters a solid tumour a little fluid can be aspirated for cytological diagnosis.

Ultrasound

Ultrasonic studies are used in many aspects of diagnostic surgery. In urological work a particular use is in the distinction between a cyst and a carcinoma of the kidney. The ultrasound study shows diffuse echoes in a solid tumour. There is a clear interface between kidney and a cyst and there are no echoes.

Cystoscopy

One of the most valuable forms of endoscopy is used for examination of the interior of the bladder. This examination is called cystoscopy. The operation is carried out in the operating room under a local, regional or general anaesthetic. After passing the instrument the bladder is emptied and then filled with glycine solution which allows a clear view. Using a fibreoptic light for illumination, the interior of the bladder can be examined in detail. Cystoscopy is used to diagnose and take biopsy specimens of tumours of the bladder. It is also used in many other cases as a part of the diagnostic study.

In addition to examination of the bladder the instrument is used to study the urethra as it is passed into the bladder. The details of prostatic enlargement can be observed.

Urinary Stones

Although a lot is known about the causes of urinary stone there is still controversy about many aspects and the cause of the most common, calcium oxalate stone, still remains obscure. In certain areas of the world there is a very high incidence of renal stones and the reason for this also remains a mystery.

Stones Forming in Sterile Urine

Stones made from uric acid or the amino acid cystine are very rare. They occur in sterile urine and are due to metabolic abnormality. The amino acid cystine is filtered in the glomerular filtrate but is not reabsorbed in the tubules and this results in an excess appearing in the urine. As water is absorbed the crystals of cystine come out of solution and may form a stone.

Calcium oxalate stones are the most common seen in patients with sterile urine. In a few cases these stones may be associated with a tumour of the parathyroid gland which causes the secretion of an excess of the hormone parathormone. Parathormone releases calcium from bones so that there is a high level of calcium in the blood and urine and this predisposes to the formation of calcium-containing stones in the kidney. However, in most cases of calcium oxalate stone there is no such abnormality. A high intake of oxalates has been incriminated and patients are usually advised to avoid eating spinach, strawberries and rhubarb because of their high oxalate content, but this is clearly not the whole story.

Stones Forming in Infected Urine

Urine normally contains urea. Certain organisms which commonly cause infection in the urinary tract produce an enzyme which acts on urea and converts it to ammonia. Ammonia alkalinises the urine so that phosphate crystals are precipitated and often form a stone by depositing on some fragment of inflammatory debris.

Clinical Effects of Stone

1   If a stone forms and grows in the kidney it may not cause any symptoms. Such a stone may grow in the pelvis and calyces of the kidney eventually filling most of the space. Because of its shape it is called a staghorn calculus. As the stone enlarges it gradually destroys the kidney and if it is bilateral the patient may present with renal failure.

2   Renal colic is one of the most severe pains which can be endured. If the stone is lodged at the junction of the renal pelvis and ureter, violent contractions of the muscle of the renal pelvis will try to get rid of the stone down the ureter. Very severe pain is felt in the loin, radiating to the iliac fossa. As the stone passes down the ureter the severe pain recurs in attacks of colic and as the stone reaches the lower end of the ureter the pain is referred to the penis and testis. A stone less than 5 mm in diameter has a chance of reaching the bladder but a stone in excess of 5 mm will almost certainly be held up in the ureter and will obstruct the kidney causing hydronephrosis, which is a condition in which the renal pelvis and calyces are dilated.

3   An infection in the urine may be the cause of a phosphate stone. In some other cases, when the stone is causing obstruction, an infection may occur as a result of stagnation of the flow of urine.

Treatment of Renal Colic

Patients with renal colic are often admitted to hospital as an acute surgical emergency. The pain is very severe and the patient may cry out during the spasms. Remember that he really is suffering very severe pain and is unable to stop rolling about in agony. The usual drug for relief of pain is an injection of pethidine which controls pain and relieves muscle spasm. The diagnosis can be confirmed with a plain X-ray of the abdomen as most renal stones contain sufficient calcium to be radio-opaque. A sample of urine should also be examined because a trace of blood is usually present in cases of renal colic.

As soon as the acute attack has subsided a urogram is ordered to identify the exact position of the stone and the degree of obstruction and function of the affected kidney.

Operations for Renal and Ureteric Stones

Stones in the kidney are usually removed. Even large staghorn stones can be removed in pieces through an incision in the kidney pelvis and sometimes in the kidney substance as well. The operation of removal of stones through the pelvis of the kidney is called pyelolithotomy. Removal through an incision in the kidney is called nephro-lithotomy.

Small stones in the kidney, less than 5 mm in diameter, are treated conservatively for a time provided the obstruction is not complete making permanent renal damage likely. X-rays taken at intervals may show that the stone has moved or even disappeared. Surprisingly patients do not always know that they have passed a stone in the urine. If a stone remains in the ureter it has to be removed. This can be done through an incision on the abdominal wall.

After removal of a stone from the kidney or ureter the opening is closed with catgut sutures. Urine nearly always leaks through the suture line so a drain is left in the wound and connected to a sterile drainage bag. Provided there is no obstruction to the ureter lower down a urinary leak or fistula will always close in a few days and the tube can be removed.

A small stone in the lower third of the ureter is sometimes removed with an instrument called a Dormia basket. This is introduced into the bladder with a cystoscope and then guided into the ureter. If it can be negotiated past the stone it is opened to catch the stone and pull it out.

Bladder Stones

If a stone is small enough to negotiate the passage from the kidney down the ureter to the bladder it is likely to be small enough to be passed with the urine. If the stone is too large it will remain in the bladder and gradually increase in size. Outflow obstruction such as prostatic enlargement may prevent passage of a stone.

A stone in the bladder often produces dramatic symptoms as it rests on the trigone, which is very sensitive and causes severe pain referred to the tip of the penis. When the patient passes urine the pain is worse and there is often some haematuria caused by the stone damaging the trigone of the bladder.

Bladder stones are removed through the urethra. The stone is crushed with a special instrument called a lithotrite and the fragments washed out. Confirmation that the fragments have all been removed is made by looking into the bladder with an endoscope.

Kidney Tumours

Most tumours of the kidney are malignant and comprise:

1   Carcinoma of the renal tubules. This is now correctly called carcinoma of the kidney but some surgeons still refer to it as a hypernephroma, which is inaccurate, or a Grawitz tumour after one of the early surgeons to describe its clinical features.

2   The lining of the urinary tract is the same from the calyces to the bladder and is called the urothelium. It is subject to the same tumours throughout its length but they are less common in the kidney than in the bladder. The usual tumour of the renal pelvis is a transitional cell carcinoma of varying degrees of malignancy. Sometimes the lining undergoes a change which is called metaplasia and as a result of this the tumour may be a squamous cell carcinoma.

3   Nephroblastoma is an embryonic tumour arising from primitive renal cells and presenting in infancy. Some surgeons call this a Wilms' tumour after a surgeon who described it in 1899.

Carcinoma of the Kidney

This tumour arises at all ages but is more common at advanced years. It is of extremely variable malignancy and may lie almost dormant for many years. The usual presentation is with painless haematuria which brings the patient to investigation. The diagnosis is usually confirmed by urography which shows a lump in the kidney displacing and deforming the calyces. The tumour tends to spread early into the veins and may actually grow through the renal vein into the inferior vena cava. Fragments of tumour breaking off the main mass give rise to secondary deposits of tumour in the lungs. Bone secondaries are also common. Local spread to adjacent viscera in the abdomen may make a carcinoma of the kidney inoperable.

Treatment. The main treatment is removal of the whole kidney (nephrectomy). This may be done through a loin or an abdominal incision. The wound is often drained.

Following recovery from the operation the patient is usually sent for postoperative X-ray therapy.

Carcinoma of the Renal Pelvis

The clinical presentation is also with haematuria. Confirmation of the diagnosis is by urography which shows the filling defect in the pelvis of the kidney. The treatment is by nephrectomy. Because of the possibility of recurrence in the retained ureter it is customary to remove the ureter at the same operation. This operation is called nephroureterectomy.

Nephroblastoma

This tumour presents in infancy. However, haematuria is an uncommon feature and in most cases the mother finds a large lump in the loin and at the same time notices that her baby is not doing well.

The treatment is by nephrectomy. In the days when this was the only treatment the prognosis was very bad and the diagnosis almost a sentence of death. Nephrectomy is now followed by a combination of radiotherapy and combination chemotherapy which has transformed the outlook.

Bladder Tumours

Although there is a great range of malignancy, all bladder tumours are now regarded as malignant. Some appear as fragile, fronded papillary tumours which have all the appearances of innocence. At the other extreme there are tumours which are solid and infiltrating.

Surgeons and pathologists stage bladder tumours to try to identify the best treatment for growths at different stages of development and spread. Tumours are said to be of stage T1 to T4. A T1 tumour is confined to the surface and is the earliest stage. There is difficulty in distinguishing between T2 and T3 as the dividing level is half the depth of the wall of the bladder which is difficult to assess clinically. A T4 tumour has extended beyond the bladder and is attached to the surrounding structures. Tumours in stage T1 and T2 have good prospects of cure but only palliative treatment can be given to tumours in the more advanced stages.

The outstanding clinical feature of bladder cancer is blood in the urine (haematuria). There are often no other signs that anything is wrong and if the haematuria is intermittent the patient may be led to believe that nothing is seriously wrong. Nothing could be further from the truth and painless haematuria is always an indication for full investigation.

Investigations

1   Urine examination may show blood to be present. Sometimes a specimen is sent for cytology. This means that the urine is examined for malignant cells which come from a cancer of the urinary tract.

2   Excretion Urography.   In the film showing bladder a filling defect representing the tumour may be shown. If the tumour is blocking a ureteric orifice there may be dilatation of the ureter on that side, or if the obstruction is complete the kidney will not show at all because it is non-functioning.

3   The crucial examination is cystoscopy under a general or regional anaesthetic. The cystoscope allows the surgeon to inspect the interior of the bladder and a tumour can easily be seen and a biopsy taken.

Treatment

Early tumours in stage T1 and T2 are treated by excision with the transurethral resectoscope. A catheter is left in the bladder at the end of the operation to prevent clot retention. The more advanced tumours may be partially removed and then treated with X-ray therapy. Removal of the whole bladder is called cystectomy. It is not often advised at the present time.

Following cystectomy the surgeon is left with the problem of the

ureters which are draining urine. At one time these were sutured to
the skin but it proved impossible to catch the urine and patients were
always wet. The ureters are now joined to an isolated piece of small
intestine and this is brought out like an ileostomy. This is sometimes
called an ileal conduit (Fig. 74).

Urostomy Bag

A stoma which discharges urine is called a urostomy and is fitted with
a urine stoma bag. There are certain differences from the ileostomy
stoma bag as the urine bag must be designed to contain liquid urine
without risk of leakage. This is achieved by an inkwell design which is
illustrated (Fig. 74). There is also a dependent outlet controlled with a
tap. This tap can be opened to empty the urine into the toilet. There is
also a tube connection so that the urostomy bag can be connected to a
large urine bag which can be used at night. After use the extension
tube is washed with water and then rinsed with an antiseptic such as
domestic bleach at a concentration of one teaspoonful to a litre of
water, and then rinsed again with tap water.

The Prostate Gland

Benign Enlargement of the Prostate Gland

Enlargement of the prostate usually begins after the age of 40 but only
a small proportion of men are seriously affected as a result. The
enlargement is probably a consequence of a change in hormone
environment and begins as a generalised increase in size with nodules
which later become more distinct and are often called adenomas. As
the enlargement proceeds the urethra is compressed from side to side
by what are called the lateral lobes. An additional projection into the
bladder is called the middle lobe. Compression of the urethra causes a
gradually increasing obstruction to the outflow of urine. There are a
number of consequences of this gradual obstruction of the prostatic
urethra (Fig. 75).

1   As the bladder has to work harder to expel urine through the
narrow urethra the muscle increases in size (hypertrophy) in the same
way that a weightlifter increases the size of his biceps by training.

2   As the obstruction proceeds the bladder fails to expel all the
urine and what remains in the bladder is called 'residual urine'. As the

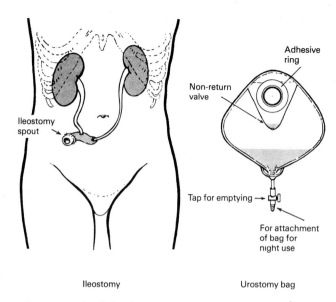

Ileostomy

Urostomy bag

Fig 74 Reconstruction following cystectomy

bladder is never completely emptied the patient feels he wants to pass urine and complains of frequency, which may be very disturbing at night. Eventually, when the bladder is very distended with residual urine, it will dribble through the sphincters causing incontinence.

3   The increasing pressure inside the bladder which results from the hypertrophied muscle may push out a part of the lining of the bladder between the muscle fibres. This begins as a little pouch and gradually grows in size to form a diverticulum of the bladder. When the patient passes urine, some passes out through the urethra and some into the diverticulum. When micturition is completed the urine in the diverticulum flows back into the bladder contributing to residual urine. Stagnation of urine in the bladder in this way sometimes results in an infection in the bladder.

4   Renal damage occurs when the obstruction is longstanding. The ureters are partly obstructed by the hypertrophied bladder muscle and dilatation of the ureters and kidneys are seen on the urogram. This is called hydroureter and hydronephrosis. The retention of waste products caused by interference with renal function causes the serious condition of uraemia.

5   Some patients suddenly get acute retention of urine. This often results from allowing the bladder to get overfilled. The large bladder obstructs the venous return from the prostate which becomes

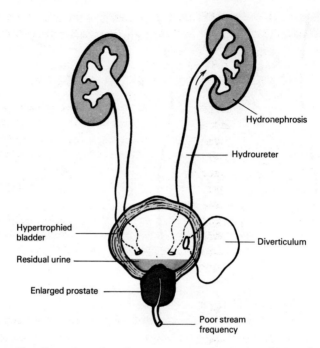

Fig 75 The effects of an enlarged prostate causing obstruction of the outflow from the bladder

congested and precipitates complete obstruction to the urethra. Acute retention of urine is a surgical emergency.

Treatment of Benign Enlargement of the Prostate Gland

The prostate gland can be removed in two ways:

1   An incision is made just above the pubes and deepened to reach the prostate behind the pubic bone. The capsule of the gland is incised and the enlargement enucleated (Millin's prostatectomy).

2   The second technique which is increasingly used in urological units is to do a transurethral resection. In this operation a special instrument called a resectoscope is passed through the penis. The instrument is used to cut strips of tissue from the prostate until it has been completely removed. The lack of an abdominal incision makes this operation easier and safer for the patient but requires special skill in the use of the resectoscope.

At the end of the open operation a drain is left in the wound. After both operations a Foley catheter is left in the bladder. Modern catheters are made of PVC or silicone. PVC is non-irritant and is perfectly suitable for use after prostectomy. Silicone is even more inert but is expensive and is reserved for patients who will need up to six weeks catheter drainage. The size of the balloon and catheter are marked on the catheter and wrapping. Catheters are marked in the French or Charrière scale which is the circumference of the catheter in millimetres.

The Foley catheter has an inflatable balloon which holds it in the bladder (Fig. 76). It is connected to a closed drainage bag.

In some hospitals an irrigation system is set up as a routine but in others it is used only when bleeding is marked. In the irrigating technique the catheter is connected to a 3-way tube (Fig. 76). A 3-litre bag of glycine irrigating fluid is hung from the drip stand and connected to one arm of the 3-way connection. Fluid is run into the bladder and then by closing the tap on the irrigation line and opening the tap on the line to the bag the fluid is run out of the bladder. The object of irrigation is to remove blood from the bladder and prevent the formation of clot which will obstruct the catheter.

Early Postoperative Management of Prostatectomy

The main early complication of the operation is continued bleeding from the prostate bed. The amount of bleeding is observed from the colour of the urine in the bag. The pulse rate and blood pressure are observed at 15 minute intervals and if the patient loses too much blood the pulse rate will rise and blood pressure fall. This calls for the replacement of blood by transfusion and also for measures to stop the bleeding. The catheter can be put under traction by pinning it to Elastoplast on the thigh, so pulling the catheter bag into the cavity of the prostate. If bleeding continues to be serious the patient may be returned to the operating room for control of the bleeding.

In most cases bleeding is insignificant and lessens quickly. The amount of fluid used for the irrigation is measured and deducted from the amount in the drainage bag to find the volume of urine secreted. Glycine is used as the irrigating fluid because it is isotonic. If water is used there is a risk that it will enter the blood stream through the open blood vessels in the prostate wound leading to haemolysis of the blood and overloading the circulation with fluid which in an elderly subject may cause heart failure.

Catheter Toilet

The meatus of the urethra tends to get inflamed and ulcerated as a result of infection with local bacteria and the presence of the catheter

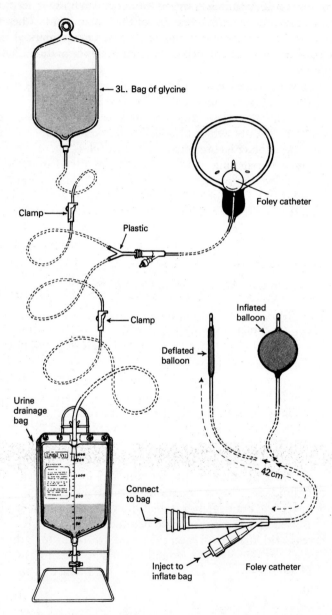

Fig 76 Bladder irrigation system

which is a foreign body. Twice daily toilet keeps the infection under control and is designed to prevent infection ascending into the bladder and prostatic bed. The area is cleansed with soapy water and then an antiseptic applied. A useful product is Lignocaine gel BPC which combines a local anaesthetic with 2 % chlorhexidine.

Catheter Fixation

The bag prevents the catheter from coming out of the bladder but the weight of tubing connecting the catheter to the drainage bag causes discomfort. This can be avoided by fixing the catheter or adjacent part of the drainage tube to the thigh. A piece of Elastoplast is fixed to the thigh and a second piece encircles the catheter. The two can then be joined together with a safety pin which must not pass through the catheter.

Later Management and Complications

The urethral catheter is generally removed about the 3rd or 4th day when bleeding has become slight.

A number of patients complain of some difficulty with control when the catheter is removed but a very small number are permanently incontinent. No satisfactory incontinence appliance has been designed for the female but a rubber drainage sheath fixed over the penis keeps the male patient dry.

Infection sometimes causes problems. The drainage system is never broken because this is an obvious way in which infection from the ward air can enter the drainage system and spread to the urinary tract. In spite of this, urinary tract infection sometimes occurs. A urine sample can be secured by opening the tap at the bottom of the bag. Antibacterial treatment is given on the basis of the results of culture of the urine in the laboratory.

Acute epididymitis may occur about a week after prostatectomy. In this case the infection reaches the epididymis along the lumen of the vas. Some surgeons routinely divide the vas at the end of the prostactectomy to prevent this complication.

Acute Retention of Urine

Sometimes a patient with enlargement of the prostate is admitted as an acute surgical emergency because he is absolutely unable to pass any urine. As the bladder fills and overfills with urine, pain becomes very severe and the bladder has to be drained.

The easiest route for relief of urinary retention is by the passage of a catheter into the bladder through the urethra. This is a sterile operation and is called aseptic catheterisation. Careless technique resulting in the introduction of infection at the very outset of treatment is nothing short of a disaster. The urethra can be anaesthetised with 1 % lignocaine jelly which is introduced into the urethra and then massaged back along the penile urethra. A small Foley catheter is selected and the end of the bag opened. The tip of the catheter is lubricated with chlorhexidine and glycerin, which is also an antiseptic. The catheter is not removed from the bag but introduced into the urethra direct from the bag with the surgeon holding and guiding the catheter by holding it through the bag. Once the catheter reaches the bladder, urine begins to drain to the great relief of the patient. It is immediately connected to a drainage bag and the balloon inflated with sterile water or saline.

If the surgeon is unable to pass a catheter into the bladder through the urethra a second route is employed. For this the patient is taken to the operating theatre and a tube introduced into the bladder through the lower abdomen just above the symphysis pubis. This is done under local anaesthetic using a balloon catheter with a steel introducer in the lumen. The instrument is introduced into the bladder and the introducer removed. The procedure is then exactly the same as with a urethral catheter. The balloon is inflated and the catheter connected to a drainage bag.

Once a catheter is in the bladder the emergency is over and the patient can be investigated at leisure with an intravenous urogram and estimation of the blood urea and electrolytes. If the blood urea and renal function are shown to be normal the patient can be treated by prostatectomy on the next available operating list providing there are no cardiac or other contraindications.

However, if the renal function is shown to be impaired the operation is deferred and catheter drainage continued until renal function returns to normal. The patient can then be treated by prostatectomy.

Carcinoma of the Prostate

Carcinoma of the prostate becomes increasingly common as age advances. It causes enlargement of the prostate and may present with the same outflow obstruction symptoms as occur in benign enlargement. It forms a hard enlargement of the prostate and the surgeon is alerted to the diagnosis when he feels the prostate on rectal examination. The cancer spreads outside the gland capsule and also spreads by the blood and lymphatic vessels. Secondary deposits are found in the pelvic lymphatic nodes. Metastases spreading into the veins often pass through the veins in front of the vertebral column and metastases develop in the lumbar and dorsal spine causing back pain.

Diagnosis

The diagnosis can sometimes be confirmed by estimation of an enzyme called acid phosphatase which is normally secreted by prostate cells. Provided the cells of the cancer are functioning, they will also produce acid phosphatase and this will cause an increase in the level in the blood. An X-ray of the spine may show secondary deposits which have a characteristic sclerotic appearance with an excess of dense new bone formed as a reaction to the cancer cells in the bone.

The final confirmation of diagnosis of any tumour is by examination of tissue from the tumour. This can often be done using the resectoscope to remove a part of the enlarged prostate for histological examination in the laboratory.

A Franzen needle can also be introduced into the prostate where the gland bulges into the rectum. A small amount of fluid is aspirated and sent for examination of the cells (cytology).

Treatment

The main line of treatment is hormone therapy as the growth is hormone dependent. Stilboestrol is given as the first treatment but urologists have not agreed about the most appropriate dose which varies from 1 to 5 mg three times daily. Unfortunately stilboestrol upsets many patients causing nausea and vomiting. Retention of fluid is a more dangerous effect and the increase in blood volume throws a strain on the heart which may induce cardiac failure or a coronary thrombosis. If these problems appear the stilboestrol is stopped and a bilateral orchidectomy (castration) advised. This has a similar effect on the cancer without the unfortunate side effects of stilboestrol.

Although the operation of total prostatectomy is often performed in the United States it is rarely performed in this country. A resection as for benign enlargement may be necessary if the patient is having great difficulty in passing urine because of compression of the urethra where it passes through the prostate.

25

The Testicle

Undescended Testicle

The testicle develops at the back of the abdomen and descends to occupy its normal position in the scrotum just before birth. Failure of this descent results in the condition of undescended testicle. The importance of non-descent lies in the fact that the testis does not function properly at the temperature which exists inside the body and normal spermatazoa are produced only at the lower temperature which exists when the testis is in the scrotum just under the skin.

The undescended testicle is treated surgically at about the age of 5 years. Later operation is somewhat easier but the risk of a non functioning testicle outweighs this disadvantage.

Torsion of the Testicle (Fig. 77 A to C)

Torsion means twisting and it is not possible in a normally placed testicle. However, if the testicle is not fixed properly in the scrotum it may hang by the spermatic cord which can easily twist causing severe pain in the testicle and cutting off the blood supply. Early surgery is essential to untwist the cord and restore the blood supply to the testicle. It is usual to explore the opposite testicle at the same operation because the anatomical abnormality is likely to be the same and torsion on the other side may occur at any time.

Hydrocoele (Fig. 77 D)

There is normally a small amount of fluid surrounding the testicle and contained in a sac called the tunica vaginalis. In some cases there is an increase in the amount of this fluid which may be very considerable. This is called an idiopathic hydrocoele because the cause is unknown. In a small number of cases the hydrocoele is secondary to disease such as a tumour in the testis and this is called a secondary hydrocoele.

A hydrocoele can be treated by aspiration of the fluid using a small bleb of local anaesthetic in the scrotal skin. This is suitable for only elderly patients who are poor operative risks as recurrence of the

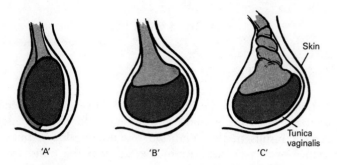

'A' shows the normal position of the testicle in the scrotum and 'B' the
abnormal position which makes torsion shown in 'C' possible

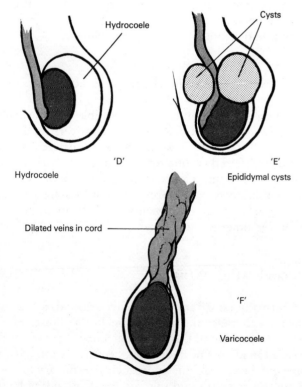

Fig 77 Surgery of the testicle

hydrocoele is inevitable and tapping will be required every few months. Most cases are treated by an operation which prevents recollection of the fluid without interference with the testicle.

Epididymal Cyst (Fig. 77 E)

Elderly patients may also complain of enlargement of the testicle which is caused by a cyst of the epididymis. Cysts may be multiple and are often bilateral. If the size proves an inconvenience the patient is treated by an operation in which the cyst and the part of the epididymis from which it is arising are removed.

Varicocoele (Fig. 77 F)

The spermatic cord contains the vas which carries spermatazoa from the testis and the testicular artery which delivers arterial blood to the testis. The main bulk of the cord consists of veins which carry blood back from the testis. Varicocoele is a condition of varicosity comparable to varicose veins in the leg. It nearly always occurs on the left side and its only known effect is that there is reduction of sperm production on that side. Surgical excision of a varicocoele is recommended in cases of male subfertility in which the sperm count is found to be reduced. Symptoms such as dragging discomfort do not merit surgical intervention which is usually followed by a complaint of similar symptoms.

Tumours of the Testicle

There are two tumours of the testicle and both are malignant.

The teratoma occurs between the ages of 20 and 30 years and the seminoma, which arises in the tubules in the testis, has its highest incidence between the ages of 30 and 40 years.

These tumours spread by the lymphatic vessels and secondary deposits of tumour occur in the para-aortic lymphatic nodes. Blood stream spread also takes place causing widespread metastases especially in the lungs in the later stages of the disease.

A tumour of the testis is treated by removal of the testicle (orchidectomy). Radiotherapy is given to the para-aortic nodes. The prognosis for patients treated for seminoma is excellent but patients with teratoma have a less good prognosis.

Postoperative Care of Scrotal Operations

The lax tissues and dependent position tend to result in a collection of blood and fluid in the scrotum after any operation. Most surgeons employ a drain and this is often a suction drain. A scrotal support helps to prevent swelling and this is best put on at the end of the operation as it may be painful to fit after recovery from the anaesthetic.

Scrotal operations are usually done through a scrotal incision. The scrotum tends to invert when sutured and many surgeons use a subcutaneous suture of absorbable material such as Dexon. This obviates the problem of removing sutures which may be difficult to see because of the skin inversion.

26

The Penis

The anatomy and physiology of the penis is described in the section on the male genital organs (page 239).

Phimosis

At birth the foreskin or prepuce is usually still adherent to the glans penis. It is not abnormal for the foreskin to be nonretractile at birth and there is no medical justification for routine circumcision in the first few days of life. Indeed it can be a very troublesome operation. Urine contains urea which is converted by bacterial action to ammonia in the baby's napkin. This is a common cause of napkin rash and the meatus of the urethra is protected by the foreskin from what is in fact an ammonia burn. Circumcision exposes the urethral orifice to the ammonia and a burn of the delicate urethral mucosa may result. This forms an ulcer which scabs and causes pain and difficulty with micturition. Although permanent trouble is unusual it is an unnecessary infliction on a helpless baby.

Phimosis is defined as a condition of nonretraction of the foreskin but it cannot be diagnosed before the age of about five years by which time the foreskin should retract.

Balanitis is an infection in the space between the foreskin and the glans. It usually occurs in a man with a nonretractile foreskin which prevents free drainage. Balanitis is a common complication of diabetes. A drop of urine containing sugar in this space provides an excellent culture medium for bacteria.

Circumcision

Circumcision is indicated for phimosis and for balanitis. Even in children, it is better to stay in hospital for a few days. Adults are certainly better treated as inpatients. The operation can be done under local anaesthetic but most surgeons prefer a general anaesthetic. After excision of the foreskin the two layers of the foreskin are sutured together at the base of the glans. No dressing is used but the area is dusted with an antibiotic powder. To avoid the difficulty of removing the sutures absorbable sutures such as catgut or Dexon are often used. There is usually a lot of swelling at the operation site but this subsides in a few days. In young men there is a danger that an erection will be very painful and many surgeons give diazepam by mouth for a few days.

Carcinoma of the Penis

Carcinoma of the penis is a rare form of carcinoma arising on the covering of the glans. It never occurs in circumcised men and it is supposed that the normal secretion produced under the foreskin which is called smegma must be carcinogenic. This means that it is a substance which causes cancer. Lack of cleanliness is also a factor in uncircumcised men.

The two available treatments are amputation of part or whole of the penis according to the extent of the disease or radiotherapy. The early cases are usually treated by radiotherapy as the results of surgery and radiation are equivalent and radiotherapy gives a better functional result. Advanced cases do not give a good response to radiotherapy and are usually treated by amputation.

27

Vascular Surgery

Surgery of Atherosclerosis

Atherosclerosis is a diffuse disease of the arteries though some arteries are more affected than others. It is a disease of affluent societies and is more common in men. One factor is probably the higher proportion of animal fat consumed by the more affluent and cigarette smoking is undoubtedly a causative factor. Some people have a higher than normal level of lipids in the blood and these patients have a high incidence of atherosclerosis which tends to come on at an early age. There is a rise in the blood fats after taking an excess of alcohol and although moderate drinking is probably harmless the heavy drinker is more likely to suffer from atherosclerosis. Diebetes mellitus is also an aetiological factor and atherosclerosis is one of the serious complications of diabetes.

The first sign of atheroma is a yellow plaque which is deposited in the inner layer of the artery (intima). As this plaque grows it begins to narrow the artery and causes turbulence in the flow of blood. Platelets from the blood are deposited on the growing plaque which eventually occludes the lumen of the artery. Once this happens the flow of blood is arrested and because of the lack of flow the blood clots for a variable distance above and below the point of the original occlusion. Gradual narrowing of the artery takes place over a period of years and as the flow diminishes other blood vessels develop to carry the blood. These are called collaterals (Fig. 78) and they may carry enough blood to compensate fully for the reduction of blood flow in the main artery. However, in most cases the collaterals are inadequate to compensate fully for the narrowing or complete occlusion and the part suffers from a reduced blood supply which is called chronic ischaemia. Chronic ischaemia affects the heart muscle as a result of narrowing of the coronary arteries. During exercise the heart has to work harder to provide more oxygenated blood for the working muscles. If the coronary arteries are narrow the additional blood cannot reach the heart muscle and the patient complains of severe chest pain which is called angina pectoria. Exactly the same thing happens when the atheromatous obstruction occurs in the arteries to the lower limb. When the patient tries to walk quickly or to run the leg muscles need more blood and the cardiac output

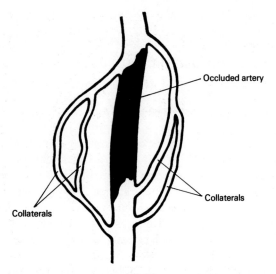

Fig 78   Collaterals developed to compensate an occlusion

increases to provide the extra oxygenated blood. If the main artery to
the leg is blocked the additional blood cannot reach the leg and the
patient complains of cramp-like pain in the muscles called intermittent claudication. In both angina pectoris and intermittent claudication the pain quickly disappears when the patient stops exercising.

Atherosclerosis is liable to cause serious trouble at certain sites:

1   the abdominal aorta and leg arteries;

2   the coronary arteries;

3   the cerebral circulation. This may be due to disease in the
arteries inside the skull or the internal carotid artery in the neck;

4   atheroma at the origin of the renal artery causes chronic renal
ischaemia and renal failure.

Acute ischaemia is a sudden arrest of the circulation to a part of the
body which may be sufficient to cause death of that part. Death of
tissue is called necrosis but in parts of the body which are exposed to
bacteria the dead muscle gets infected and the condition is called
gangrene. Gangrene of the leg can also be caused by chronic
ischaemia which has progressed to the stage at which there is
insufficient blood flow at rest to sustain life in the leg.

Atherosclerosis of the Arteries to the Legs

It can be seen from the diagram showing the anatomy of the arteries
(Fig. 79) that narrowing or occlusion of the abdominal aorta will

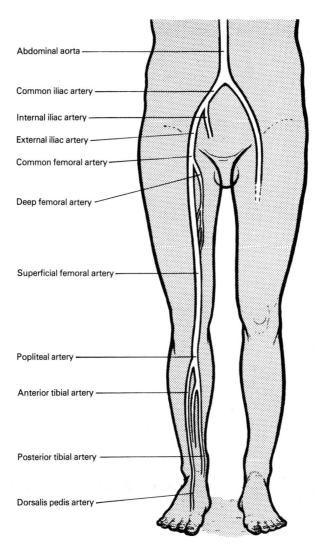

Fig 79 Anatomy of leg arteries

cause chronic ischaemia in both legs and that narrowing or occlusion of any of the arteries below the aorta will cause chronic ischaemia on the same side. The symptoms of chronic ischaemia are:

1 **Intermittent Claudication.** When the disease affects the aorta or iliac arteries the claudication pain is felt in the buttock muscles and sometimes in the thigh or calf. The most common site for intermittent claudication is the calf muscle and this is usually due to

occlusion of the superficial femoral artery. Occlusion of the arteries below the knee causes pain on walking in the muscles of the sole of the foot – plantar claudication.

Intermittent claudication may be very mild and a very slight disability but it is always serious because it indicates that the patient has atherosclerosis which is a generalised disease of the arteries. Many patients with intermittent claudication die from acute cardiac ischaemia caused by a coronary artery thrombosis. In some cases the pain is severe and incapacitating and it may prevent a man from doing his job.

2   **Rest pain** is a symptom of more severe ischaemia caused by reduced blood supply to the nerve endings. At an earlier stage there is a complaint of numbness or abnormal sensations such as pins and needles which are called paraesthaesia. Later this is replaced by severe constant pain which prevents sleep and is difficult to relieve with drugs. Severe rest pain is a symptom which demands some form of treatment.

3   **Gangrene.**   In the most severe form of chronic ischaemia the blood flow to the toes or foot is insufficient to sustain life and gangrene develops. This is nearly always accompanied by rest pain.

Investigations of Vascular Patients

As the disease is generalised some investigations are directed to cardiac and renal function. Most patients will have an electrocardiogram and a urine examination to exclude diabetes. Some surgeons also ask for an estimation of the blood lipids.

Arteriography

The particular test used in vascular cases is arteriography which gives an exact X-ray picture of the site and extent of the vascular disease. The test is done in the X-ray department. Atherosclerotic arteries may undergo patchy calcification but apart from this they are not shown on ordinary X-rays. The principle of the test is that a non-toxic radio-opaque material is injected into the artery. X-ray photographs taken after the injection will show the lumen of the artery and any occlusions. The blood flow in an artery is very rapid and special mechanical techniques are used to take a series of pictures moving down the leg at approximately the same speed as the blood flow. In most centres the injection is given into the abdominal aorta so that a complete picture of the arteries of both legs is obtained, so enabling the surgeon to have the maximum data on which to base his decision concerning the type of reconstruction which is needed. There are two techniques for the introduction of the radio-opaque material into the aorta:

1 **Translumbar Aortography (TLA).** This investigation is performed under a general anaesthetic with the patient in the prone position. The radiologist introduces a long needle into the abdominal aorta. The aorta is a large artery and it is generally easy to puncture by this technique. Successful puncture is indicated by the pulsatile flow of blood from the needle. Following recovery from the anaesthetic the patient is returned to the ward. Lumbar aortography is not entirely without risk because many of the patients have poor cardio-respiratory function. There is an additional risk of bleeding from the puncture hole in the aorta. This usually bleeds for some time and is gradually closed with a plug of platelets. The investigation cannot be done if the patient is on anticoagulants or has any clotting defect. The important nursing observations are those necessary to detect a severe blood loss from the puncture such as a rise in the pulse rate and fall in blood pressure accompanied by sweating. If these features appear in the recovery period medical aid should be sought and blood transfusion is sometimes needed.

2 **Femoral Artery Catheterisation.** The second technique which can be used to introduce radio-opaque material into the aorta is through a plastic catheter which is introduced through the femoral artery. The femoral artery is placed superficially just below the groin crease and a catheter introduced at this point can be directed through the iliac arteries to the aorta where the injection is made. This technique is sometimes known by the name of Seldinger, who first described it. Specially shaped catheter tips can be introduced into a main branch of the aorta and in this way a selective arteriogram can be done, for example, of the renal artery.

Aortic catheterisation through the femoral artery is done with a local anaesthetic. The puncture site leaks blood after removal of the catheter but this can be minimised by local pressure with a sterile sponge for five minutes. Bleeding may recur after return to the ward and the nurse should look at the site frequently during the first six hours and apply pressure should external bleeding or haematoma occur.

All forms of arterial catheterisation may be complicated by

thrombosis of the artery or by dislodgement of a plaque of atheroma into the lumen. A sudden occlusion causes acute ischaemia. The limbs should be observed for colour and temperature changes following arteriography. Acute ischaemia also causes paralysis of the muscles and anaesthaesia of the skin on the affected leg. If there are signs of acute ischaemia the medical staff must be informed at once.

Vascular Laboratory

Large centres of vascular surgery are supported by a vascular laboratory in which tests using ultrasound are used. These tests give useful information and are non-invasive. This means that there is no need for any preparation of the patient and the study is completely safe. The patient is told that his circulation will be studied by passing a probe over the surface of the leg at the site of the main artery. Ultrasound is sound waves which are of a frequency outside the range which is audible to the human ear. The ultrasonic waves are reflected from moving red blood corpuscles and the Doppler effect observed. If the blood corpuscles are moving away the wavelength is lengthened and if they are moving towards the probe the wavelength is shortened after reflection. The reflected sound waves are picked up by the probe and converted to electrical impulses which can be recorded photographically. This technique gives a picture of the blood flowing inside the artery and therefore shows any abnormality of contour of the lining and any occlusions.

Another type of Doppler scanner called a B mode scanner can be used to show the wall of the artery or graft.

Pulse Volume Recording

Pulse volume recording is particularly used during the operation to record the pulse wave before and after the reconstruction. It is also used during postoperative observation because it is much more reliable than clinical observations as a guide to patency of the reconstruction.

A blood pressure cuff is placed on the calf of the leg. The arterial pulse wave is transferred to the air in the bag. At the end of the tube leading from the bag is a device called a transducer which converts pressure changes to electrical currents and these are electronically converted to wave forms which are recorded continuously.

Non-surgical Management of Patients with Atherosclerosis

All patients, whether to be treated by surgical reconstruction or not, should be given advice about their general management:

1 It is essential that the patient should stop smoking as this contributes to the progress of the disease.

2 Exercise may promote the development of a collateral circulation and patients should walk as far as possible within the limits of their intermittent claudication.

3 Blood abnormality, especially anaemia, must be corrected. The increased oxygen-carrying capacity of the blood which results from correction of anaemia may cause considerable improvement.

4 Anticoagulant drugs have not been shown to be of value and although vasodilator drugs are often prescribed there is no evidence that any benefit results from their use.

5 Aspirin prevents the formation of platelet thrombi on atheromatous plaques and is at present under trial.

Management of Aortoiliac Disease

Aortoiliac disease may give rise to three effects:

1 **Intermittent claudication** which may be felt in the buttock or calf.

2 **Gangrene.**   There is normally a free anastomosis between the great vessels and these usually open sufficiently to give an adequate collateral circulation. When the patient has gangrene he usually has disease in the femoral artery as well. If this is the case the proximal occlusion is treated first.

3 **Impotence.**   Disease in the aorta or common iliac artery reduces the flow of blood in the internal iliac artery and as this provides the blood flow to the pelvic organs and the penis there may be insufficient blood for the patient to get an erection. The combination of buttock claudication and impotence is called Leriche's syndrome. It is rarely improved by reconstruction.

Treatment is advised according to the severity of the symptoms. Gangrene is always an indication for reconstruction as the alternative is amputation. When claudication is severe enough to interfere with a patient's work or pleasure reconstruction is considered. Large arteries are usually reconstructed with Dacron tubes which are crimped to reduce the danger of kinking. Dacron tubes develop a lining about

2 mm in depth which is called a pseudointima because it is made of fibrin and platelets. In some centres the operation of endarterectomy is still used. In this operation, which is sometimes referred to as reboring, the artery is opened and the atheroma and thrombosis is removed. Finally the artery is closed with sutures.

Aortic Bifurcation Graft

A variety of reconstructions are done depending on the sites of the disease and the general condition of the patient. If the patient is in reasonably good general condition the aorta is transected and the end of the Dacron graft is sutured to the end of the aorta (Fig. 80). The two lower limbs of the graft may be sutured to the iliac, femoral or profunda femoris artery as indicated by the site of the obstruction which has to be bypassed.

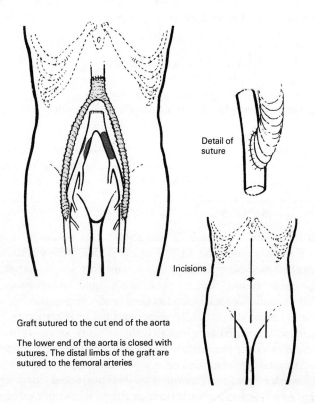

Detail of suture

Incisions

Graft sutured to the cut end of the aorta

The lower end of the aorta is closed with sutures. The distal limbs of the graft are sutured to the femoral arteries

Fig 80 Aorto-bifemoral bypass graft

Femoro-femoral Crossover Graft

When the condition of the patient is poor it is possible to do an extra-anatomical graft. This is a graft which takes a completely different route from the natural one.

The femoro-femoral crossover graft (Fig. 81) is indicated when one iliac artery is occluded and the other is normal. The operation is easy and as the arteries are superficially placed the disturbance to the patient is slight.

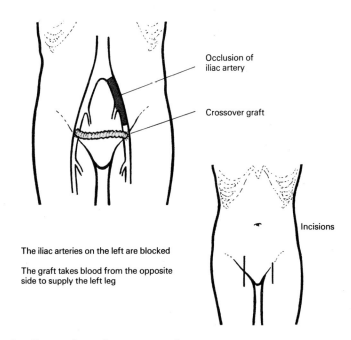

Occlusion of iliac artery

Crossover graft

Incisions

The iliac arteries on the left are blocked

The graft takes blood from the opposite side to supply the left leg

Fig 81   Femoro–femoral crossover graft

Axillo-bifemoral Graft (Fig. 82)

When there is aortoiliac disease but the patient's condition is poor it is possible to revascularise the legs by taking a long Dacron graft from the axillary artery. Although this does not carry as much blood as a graft directly from the aorta it gives a very worthwhile improvement. The graft is bifurcated so that one limb goes to each femoral artery because this increases the flow and improves the long term patency rate. Like the femoro-femoral graft this extra-anatomical graft runs subcutaneously and its insertion does not seriously disturb the patient. However, there is one serious problem with the axillofemoral graft. Because of its long subcutaneous course on the trunk it may be compressed during sleep and patients are advised not to sleep on the side of the graft because prolonged compression results in thrombosis.

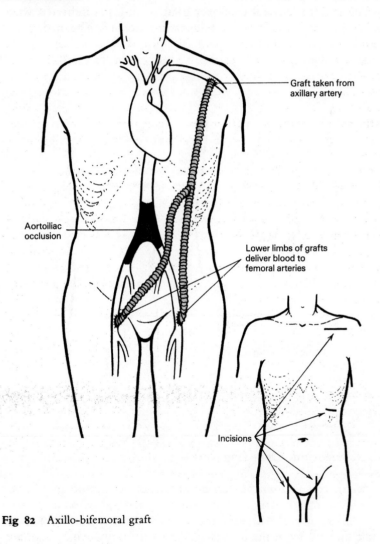

Graft taken from axillary artery

Aortoiliac occlusion

Lower limbs of grafts deliver blood to femoral arteries

Incisions

Fig 82 Axillo-bifemoral graft

Management of Femoropopliteal Disease

Atherosclerotic occlusion of the femoral or popliteal arteries usually causes more severe symptoms then aortoiliac disease. Intermittent claudication is felt in the calf of the leg and may vary from a slight inconvenience to severe and incapacing pain. Rest pain and gangrene are also seen as a result of femoropopliteal disease and are always an indication to consider a reconstruction operation. Operations for intermittent claudication are less satisfactory at this level and are not usually recommended unless the symptom is very severe.

The Dacron graft, which is so important in the treatment of aortoiliac disease, is not used in femoropopliteal reconstruction as the lower blood flow results in early thrombosis of the graft. However, the long saphenous vein is often wide enough to use as a graft and it has the advantage that it is autogenous, which means that it is from the same subject so that there will be no rejection problem. A skin graft is another example of an autograft.

If the long saphenous vein is not large enough it is possible to use other materials but nothing matches the success of a good long saphenous vein. The substitutes for a vein graft are:

1   Dardik.   This is an allograft, which means that it is a graft taken from a member of the same species, i.e. in this case a human blood vessel but from another subject. The Dardik graft is umbilical vein which has been tanned with gluteraldehyde. There is some risk of rejection which may result in dilatation and so the graft is sheathed in a mesh of polyester.

2   The second possible choice is a synthetic graft called Gore-Tex which is made from polytetrafluorethylene.

The femoropopliteal graft is not a difficult operation and blood loss is very slight. If saphenous vein is used it has to be removed through a long incision and then reversed in direction before being sutured to the femoral and popliteal arteries (Fig. 83). This is because the long saphenous vein is valved to assist the return of blood from the foot towards the heart and if the vein is not reversed the valves will obstruct the circulation. If a Dardik or Gore-Tex graft is used the operation can be done through two small incisions at each end and the graft tunnelled between the two incisions.

Profundoplasty

In some cases the arteriogram shows narrowing of the profunda femoris artery in addition to occlusion of the superficial femoral

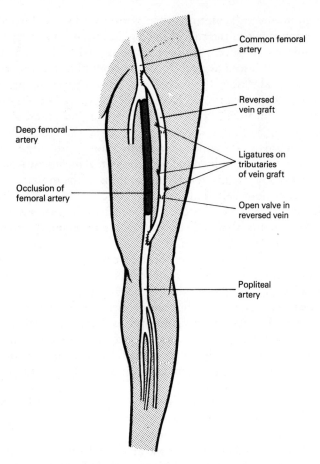

Fig 83 Femoropopliteal vein bypass graft

artery. Profundoplasty (Fig. 84) will increase the flow of blood down the profunda femoris artery and so improve the foot circulation through collaterals in the region of the knee joint.

Lumbar Sympathectomy

The principle of lumbar sympathectomy is described on page 287. Some surgeons still advise this operation but the effect on the circulation is very marginal in cases of severe ischaemia due to atherosclerosis. If lumbar sympathectomy is advised it is easier for the

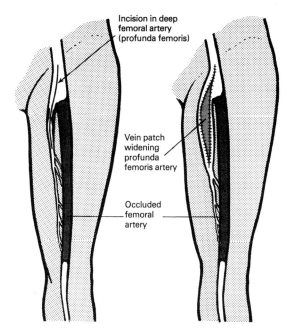

Fig 84 Profundoplasty

patient, and probably just as effective, to accomplish it by giving an injection of 6% phenol into the sympathetic nerve to destroy it chemically rather than doing an operation to remove the nerve.

Combined Iliac and Femoral Disease

When the iliac and femoral artery are both narrowed or occluded there is usually severe chronic ischaemia. Some surgeons treat this by taking a Dacron graft from the iliac artery above the occlusion and joining it to the profunda femoris artery (Fig. 85). This extra pressure in the profunda artery greatly improves the circulation in the thigh and through the collaterals round the knee joint giving an improvement in circulation to the foot which is sometimes enough to avert a thigh level amputation. A more dramatic improvement to the foot circulation is achieved by doing an ileopopliteal Dacron graft (Fig. 86). This operation transmits the high pressure iliac blood directly to the popliteal artery which carries it into the leg arteries passing to the foot. The dramatic improvement in the blood supply to the foot makes it possible to amputate any localised gangrene at the same operation.

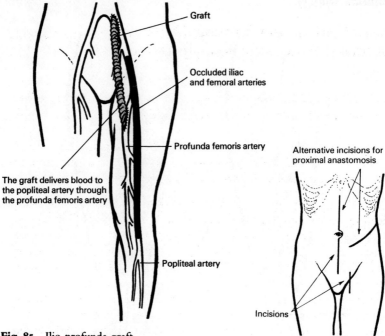

Fig 85 Ilio-profunda graft

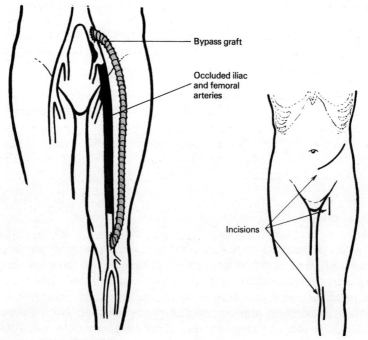

Fig 86 Iliopopliteal graft
An alternative operation for combined iliac and femoral disease

Complications and Nursing Observations following Reconstruction Operations

The two important complications of arterial reconstruction operations are bleeding from the suture line and early thrombosis of the graft.

The patient will return from the operation with suction drains and wound dressings. The Opsite dressing is very useful as the nursing staff can see the wound without exposing it to the ward air.

1   The pulse and blood pressure are taken at 15 minute intervals. Bleeding from the suture lines may be indicated by swelling caused by haematoma or by frank bleeding from the wound or from the suction drain. Blood normally clots in the tissues but vascular operations are always done with heparin anticoagulation which may still be operative in the recovery room and allow fluid blood to discharge from the drain. Haematoma and frank bleeding from the wound may be seen when the anastomosis is near the surface but if bleeding from the aortic anastomosis occurs the patient will show the generalised effects of raised pulse rate and fall in blood pressure accompanied by sweating. The doctor should be alerted if there are signs of external or internal bleeding. The management may comprise blood transfusion and correction of any residual coagulation defect but some patients may be returned to the operating room for control of the bleeding.

2   Observations on the leg. It is unusual for foot pulses to be present immediately after a reconstruction operation. The arteries below the knee are often narrow and there is also arterial spasm which contributes to the difficulty in feeling the foot pulses. Reliance has usually to be placed on the colour and temperature of the foot which should gradually become warm and pink. Clinical appraisal is often difficult in the first few hours and if it is available it is better to measure the pulse with the pulse volume recorder. Deterioration in the circulation should be reported to the surgeon.

3   Severe bleeding is unusual in modern vascular surgery but if it occurs and is accompanied by a period of hypotension there may be interference with renal function. Most cases return from the operation with a urinary catheter attached to a sterile drainage bag enabling the nurse to observe and record the urinary output. Other observations and treatment of hypovolaemic shock are described in Chapter 7.

4   The transperitoneal approach to the aorta requires retraction of the intestines during the time that the surgeon is exposing the aorta and making the anastomosis to the Dacron graft. Following this disturbance the intestines do not function for several days. This condition is called paralytic ileus and an indwelling gastric tube is required until intestinal function recovers. As the patient is unable to take and absorb fluids an intravenous infusion will also be required.

5   Patients should be able to take weight on the leg and walk a few steps on the day following the operation.

6   Many surgeons employ prophylactic antibiotics which are started about one hour before the operation. If the first dose is given with the premedication there will be an effective level of antibiotic in the blood and tissues at the time of the operation when most wound infections begin.

Cerebrovascular Disease

Anatomy of the Arteries Supplying the Brain

The brain receives its blood supply from two carotid and two vertebral arteries. Atherosclerosis affecting any of these vessels may have dramatic effects.

Carotid Arteries.   The two carotid arteries lie at the side of the neck under cover of a large muscle called the sternomastoid muscle. The right carotid arises from the innominate artery but the left carotid arises directly from the arch of the aorta. At the level of the upper border of the larynx the carotids divide into two smaller arteries called the internal and external carotid arteries. The external carotid artery remains outside the skull and its branches are distributed to the thyroid, tongue, face, scalp and jaws. The internal carotid artery passes through a foramen in the base of the skull and joins a circular system of arteries called the Circle of Willis which lies between the base of the skull and the brain. The internal carotid blood is distributed to the brain (Fig. 87).

Vertebral Arteries.   There is a vertebral artery on each side of the body. Each arises from the subclavian artery and takes an unusual course through the transverse processes of the cervical vertebrae. When it leaves the first cervical vertebra it enters the skull through the foramen magnum which is the main opening in the base of the skull through which the spinal cord is linked to the medulla oblongata of

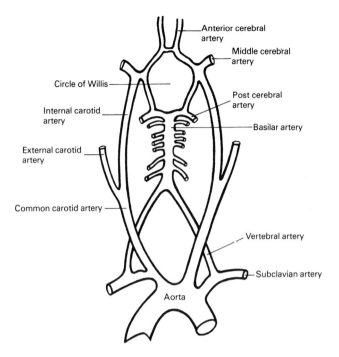

Fig 87 Anatomy of cerebral circulation

the brain. The two vertebral arteries join to form an artery called the basilar artery which runs close to and gives branches to the base of the brain which controls the vital functions of life. The basilar artery then divides into two arteries called the posterior cerebral arteries which supply the back of the brain but also communicate with the Circle of Willis (Fig. 87). The blood from all four arteries mixes in the Circle of Willis although most of the carotid blood finishes in the front and middle of the brain and the vertebral blood finishes mainly in the back of the brain. When there is narrowing of one of the four arteries it may be compensated by increase in flow of the others so that the Circle of Willis is an arterial system which protects the brain from ischaemia.

Small aneurysms sometimes form on the arteries of the Circle of Willis. They may appear at any age and their cause is not known. Unfortunately they may rupture causing damage to the brain and sudden coma. If possible these small aneurysms are treated by placing a clip across the mouth so isolating the bleeding aneurysm from its parent artery.

There is some dispute concerning the cause of cerebral symptoms which result from atherosclerosis in the cerebral circulation. When a plaque causes narrowing of an artery and reduction of blood flow it is possible that it would cause ischaemia of the brain in the same way as narrowing of the femoral artery causes ischaemia of the foot and leg. However it is likely that another mechanism is a more common cause. When an atheromatous plaque ulcerates it is soon covered by a platelet thrombus and tiny platelet emboli are now thought to be the usual cause of brain symptoms associated with carotid or vertebral atherosclerosis.

Clinical Syndromes

1   Vertebrobasilar Ischaemia.   Thrombi which form on an atheromatous ulcer at the origin of the vertebral artery pass through the basilar artery and may enter the posterior cerebral artery on either side. It is therefore difficult to localise the site of the lesion and there may be sudden attacks of numbness or weakness in the limbs. Transitory blindness, double vision (diplopia) or giddiness (vertigo) are also symptoms of minute embolus into the base of the brain or the posterior cerebral hemispheres.

2   Carotid Disease.   Atheroma usually occurs in the internal carotid artery just above its origin from the common carotid artery. Because the internal carotid blood is distributed to the brain on the same side it is easy to localise from the symptoms. Emboli cause sudden attacks of weakness and numbness in the limbs on one side of the body. The nerve tracts from the cerebral hemispheres cross in the brain and are distributed to the opposite side of the body. If the right carotid artery is affected the right side of the brain is embolised but symptoms and signs appear on the left side. Speech is usually represented in a small area of the left side of the brain so that there may be difficulty with speech (dysphasia) when the disease affects the left carotid artery. In left-handed people the speech centre is often on the right side of the brain.

It is typical of the syndrome that there are transient attacks of weakness and dysphasia with rapid recovery and these attacks are called transient ischaemic attacks (TIA).

3   The Subclavian Steal Syndrome.   The term 'steal' is used in vascular surgery when, as a result of an occlusion, blood flow takes a different route and this may result in a reduction to some other part of the body which is then said to be the subject of 'steal'.

A good example of a 'steal' syndrome occurs when there is an atherosclerotic occlusion of the origin of the left subclavian artery. The low pressure in the subclavian artery beyond the occlusion causes a reversal of blood flow in the left vertebral artery so 'stealing' blood from the basilar circulation (Fig. 88).

A variety of symptoms may result:

1   ischaemia, including gangrene, of the fingers of the same side;
2   signs of cerebral ischaemia such as dizzy attacks and vertigo;
3   a combination of brain and hand symptoms.

Investigation

The key investigation in cerebrovascular disease is arteriography. This may be done by introducing radio-opaque contrast material into the carotid artery. When the subclavian artery is involved, or more comprehensive information is needed, an arch aortogram is done. A catheter is introduced into the femoral artery at the groin and passed proximally until it reaches the arch of the aorta when the injection is given.

Treatment

In recent years there has been a division of opinion concerning the treatment. Some physicians advise the use of drugs which prevent the aggregation of platelets so preventing the formation of a platelet thrombus on the plaque. Aspirin is most commonly used for this purpose and good results are claimed.

In the hands of a good vascular surgeon many cases can be treated very successfully by operation.

Carotid Disease.   The carotid arteries are exposed and after clamping the internal carotid is opened and the atheromatous plaque removed. The artery is then sutured. Irreversible brain damage occurs if the complete brain circulation is arrested for three minutes. The time limit for clamping one internal carotid is difficult to assess and to some extent depends on the amount of disease and narrowing present in the other arteries supplying the brain which can contribute blood through the Circle of Willis. Some surgeons employ a plastic tube to bypass the part clamped during the operation.

Subclavian Steal Syndrome.   When symptoms are severe surgical treatment is indicated as there is no medical alternative. A graft is

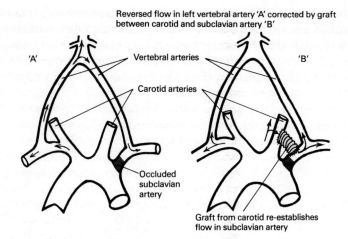

Fig 88   Subclavian steal syndrome

taken from the carotid to the subclavian beyond the occlusion. Earlier fears that this would significantly reduce the cerebral circulation through the carotids have not been substantiated (Fig. 88).

Postoperative Observations

The patient returns to the ward with a sutured wound and usually a suction drain.

As with all vascular operations some of the observations are concerned with the possibility of bleeding from the arterial suture line. This may appear as external bleeding as the artery is superficially placed. There may also be a haematoma in the neck. This carries particular danger as it may compress the trachea and cause breathing difficulty. Swelling in the neck is always an indication to call for medical aid.

The other important observations in carotid surgery are concerned with brain function. If all is well the patient will gradually regain consciousness. Failure to regain consciousness indicates serious brain damage. Other observations would include the size of the pupils and their reaction to light.

Percutaneous Transluminal Angioplasty (Fig. 89)

Transluminal angioplasty is a technique in which a balloon is passed into the narrowed atheromatous artery and inflated so increasing the size of the artery. The balloon is passed through an arterial puncture and the idea that atherosclerosis can be treated in this simple way is very attractive. The idea was first promoted in 1964 but it was not until 1974 when Grüntzig introduced the strong walled polyvinyl balloon that the technique began to gain popularity. Initially it was used to treat stenosis or occlusion in the femoral and iliac arteries but by using special catheter techniques angioplasty is now being used for stenosis of the renal and coronary arteries.

A catheter is first passed into the femoral artery at the groin and guided into the stenotic area. A guide wire is then passed through the catheter and the catheter removed leaving the guide wire in position. The Grüntzig balloon catheter is then passed over the wire which is used to guide the balloon into position. When correctly placed the balloon is inflated, so dilating the stenosis. At the time of the dilatation the artery wall is damaged allowing the projecting plaque to be displaced outwards.

It is too early to assess the place of transluminal angioplasty in the treatment of atherosclerosis but it is an attractive idea and is widely practiced in the United States at the present time.

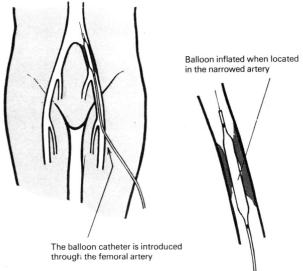

Balloon inflated when located
in the narrowed artery

The balloon catheter is introduced
through the femoral artery

Fig 89 Percutaneous transluminal angioplasty

Post Procedural Care

There is some debate about the question of anticoagulation therapy but many physicians and interventional radiologists believe that post dilatation anticoagulation is necessary. Interventional radiologist is a title now given to a radiologist who uses radiological techniques to treat patients.

The main complications of transluminal angioplasty are embolism from thrombus which forms at the site of the operation and complete arterial occlusion at the site of the dilatation caused by damage to the intimal lining of the artery. Both of these complications result in acute ischaemia of the limb and the main nursing observations are directed to observing the leg which has been treated. The sudden onset of colour changes associated with numbness suggest acute ischaemia and are an indication for the nurse to call the doctor.

Arterial Embolism

An embolus is something which travels with the blood inside the blood vessels. It is usually a thrombus or blood clot which has formed in the heart. An arterial embolus travels in the arteries which get smaller as they divide and eventually it is stopped because the artery is no longer large enough for it to pass any further. This causes a dramatic surgical emergency because the embolus causes a sudden arrest of the circulation to the part supplied by the particular artery which is blocked.

Most emboli arise in the heart. In cases of stenosis of the mitral valve the left atrium may not contract properly. Instead it has a writhing action which is called fibrillation. This causes some stagnation in the left atrium where thrombus may form and this may become detached at any time. When this happens the fragment of thrombus passes through the mitral valve into the left ventricle and is then pumped out through the aortic valve into the aorta. Only chance determines exactly where it may end but most emboli occlude an artery leading to the lower limb or actually in the leg. The bifurcation of the aorta and the division of the common femoral artery are two of the most common sites for an embolus to occur. Another type of arterial embolus occurs about seven to ten days after a myocardial infarction in which a thrombus has formed on the inside of the left ventricle where it is necrotic following a coronary artery thrombosis. In the majority of cases the pulse is irregular or there is a recent history of myocardial infarction.

Most emboli occur in the limbs, particularly the lower limb. The effect of sudden arrest of the circulation is characteristic. The patient complains that the limb suddenly became painful and very soon after its function was impaired. The colour is often white at first and then blue. The limb is cold and the pulses are absent below the point of the embolism.

The subsequent course varies according to the site of embolism and also the collateral circulation which is present. Initially the arteries of the leg go into spasm beyond the point of embolism but this soon wears off and the circulation recovers as blood reaches the distal artery through collaterals. In the worst case the ischaemia is so severe that the patient will lose the limb because of gangrene. Many cases recover enough for this tragedy to be avoided but the limb's function is permanently impaired. The severity of the ischaemia is judged from the effect it has on the peripheral nerves. If the motor nerves are not working because of ischaemia, the leg will be paralysed and if the sensory nerves are not functioning, the patient will not be able to feel light touch. If the limb is paralysed and anaesthetic the prognosis for it is indeed serious.

Within about six hours the blood begins to thrombose in the stagnant blood in the artery beyond the embolus. This is called propagated thrombus and it often makes surgical treatment more difficult in patients who are operated on after a lapse of more than six hours.

Embolism of the arteries to the brain causes a stroke because the blood supply to part of the brain is arrested. Another rare but very serious site of embolism is the origin of the superior mesenteric artery which is the branch of the abdominal aorta which supplies blood to most of the small intestine. Very few patients survive this catastrophe because the small intestine becomes necrotic. Soon after bacteria in the intestine invade the dead intestine causing putrefaction or gangrene.

Treatment of Arterial Emboli

Non-surgical Treatment

As most cases have some cardiac pathology it is often wise to seek the opinion of a cardiologist. As far as the local condition is concerned it is essential to put the patient on heparin as soon as possible. This prevents the propagation of thrombus in the artery beyond the point of the embolus and if surgery is deferred for some reason there is no added difficulty. An intravenous infusion is set up and heparin administered as a continuous infusion using an automatic clockwork device. It is usual to give 20 000 units in each 24 hours.

Surgical Treatment

The surgical operation for removal of an embolus is called embolectomy. It can generally be carried out under local anaesthetic. The artery is opened as near to the site of the embolus as is anatomically convenient and the embolus and any propagated clot are removed by passing balloon catheters. These are passed beyond the thrombus and then pulled back after inflation of the balloon (Fig. 90).

The same operation can be performed in cases of mesenteric embolism but the intestine is often gangrenous by the time the surgeon operates and there is nothing to do except a very extensive resection of small intestine.

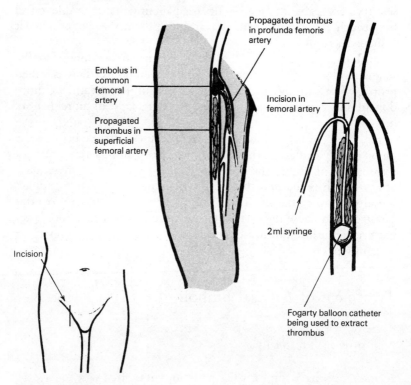

Embolus in common femoral artery

Propagated thrombus in superficial femoral artery

Propagated thrombus in profunda femoris artery

Incision in femoral artery

2 ml syringe

Incision

Fogarty balloon catheter being used to extract thrombus

Fig 90   Embolectomy

Postoperative Nursing Observations

As with any operation on an artery, there is a possibility of haemorrhage from the artery suture line, especially if the patient is heparinised. The suction drain may drain more than expected or a large lump at the wound site indicates a haematoma. The wound should be inspected frequently after the operation and the doctor called if there is evidence of bleeding. One important control in patients on heparin is the thrombin clotting time because wound bleeding may be due to an overdose of heparin.

The circulation of the leg or arm beyond the site of the operation is watched and any deterioration reported.

One unfortunate complication of this condition is that there is usually more thrombus in the heart and a further embolus in the postoperative period is quite common. Most patients are kept on long term anticoagulation to prevent reformation of thrombus in the heart.

The Sympathectic Nervous System – Sympathectomy

The sympathetic nerves are intimately connected with the rest of the nervous system. They originate in the brain and pass down the spinal cord together with the nerves destined to supply the muscles and to receive sensory impulses from the skin. The peripheral nerve trunks leave the spinal cord at every segment from one end of the cord to the other but the sympathetic nerves leave the spinal cord only in the part which includes the 12 dorsal and first two lumbar segments. After leaving the spinal cord the sympathetic nerves enter a long nerve called the sympathetic chain which runs on the front of the vertebral column from the skull to the coccyx. The nerves may pass up or down in the sympathetic chain before rejoining the peripheral nerves to be distributed to the peripheral arteries and to the sweat glands and hair follicles in the skin. A stimulus passing through the sympathetic nerves causes narrowing of the arteries, sweating and erection of the hairs.

Fear is associated with sympathetic nerve activity and causes pallor, sweating and erection of the hairs. Other sympathetic nerves do not re-enter the peripheral nerves but pass as sympathetic nerve trunks to the viscera in the chest and abdomen. The heart, lungs and all the intestines are innervated in this way.

Sympathectomy

As all the sympathetic nerves to the skin and arteries of the limbs pass through the sympathetic chain it is obvious that excision of the correct part of the chain will prevent the normal sympathetic responses. The effect of sympathectomy on the skin are:

1   dilatation of the small arteries and an increase in blood flow to the part which has been denervated;

2   sweating in the same part will be abolished.

Sympathectomy is used to increase the blood flow to a limb which is affected by chronic ischaemia. It is not generally successful if the ischaemia is due to atherosclerosis as the arteries are so rigid that dilatation is not possible. Its main indications are Buerger's disease, which is treated by lumbar sympathectomy, and Raynaud's disease, which is treated by upper dorsal sympathectomy. Upper dorsal sympathectomy is very rarely used to prevent sweating in the hands when it is so excessive that it interferes with a patient's life.

Lumbar sympathectomy is performed through an abdominal incision. The operation reflects the peritoneum and avoids entering the peritoneal cavity. This is an easy operation with good results in well selected cases and no special aftercare is needed.

Upper dorsal sympathectomy used to be called cervical sympathectomy because the operation was done through an incision in the neck just above the clavicle. Many surgeons find this operation easier by taking the direct route through the chest. An incision is made in the axilla and about four inches of the third rib excised. The lung is retracted to reach the sympathetic chain where it lies on the front of the vertebral column. There are not usually any postoperative problems with this operation but as it is a thoracotomy a drain will be left in the chest and this must be drained into a thoracotomy bottle. A chest X-ray is taken immediately after the operation and another on the second day before the tube is removed. Breathing exercises are recommended to ensure full reflation of the lung which is collapsed during the operation.

Aneurysms

An aneurysm is a dilated part of an artery caused by disease weakening the wall and causing it to stretch under the pressure of the blood. The most common cause of an aneurysm at the present time is atherosclerosis, which is also responsible for arterial occlusions. Atherosclerotic aneurysms are most commonly seen in the abdominal aorta, the popliteal and femoral arteries but no artery is exempt.

Whatever the site, all aneurysms carry the risk of bursting (ruptured or leaking aneurysm) and of throwing off emboli of blood thrombus which has formed within the sac of the aneurysm. Each of these complications has such serious consequences that surgical treatment is recommended for all aneurysms unless the condition of the patient is very poor.

Abdominal Aortic Aneurysm

Aneurysm of the abdominal aorta is the most common aneurysm seen at the present time. It becomes common after the age of 60 years and is a manifestation of atherosclerosis. It is nearly always situated in the lowest part of the aorta between the renal artery branches and the division into the two iliac arteries. This position is fortunate as the surgeon can resect the aneurysm without interference with the blood flow to the kidneys.

Rupture of an aneurysm is sudden and unexpected. If the rupture is into the peritoneal cavity death from haemorrhage follows quickly and the patient does not reach hospital. However, if the rupture is behind the peritoneum, blood leaks into the retroperitoneal tissues causing a giant haematoma. Signs of serious internal haemorrhage are obvious but although the patient collapses with hypovolaemic shock he usually survives long enough to reach the hospital emergency department. This is one of the greatest surgical emergencies and surgeons and nurses must understand that the only hope for survival is to stop the catastrophic bleeding. There is no place for attempts at resuscitation nor for the niceties of the routine preparation for theatre. The patient is transferred to the operating table as soon as the diagnosis is made and it does not matter if he or even the surgeon is not wearing the usual theatre uniform. The essence is to operate before the patient dies of haemorrhage or his kidney or brain function irreversibly fail because of prolonged hypotension. Once the surgeon has a clamp on the aorta above the aneurysm the situation is under control and the anaesthetist can run in blood until the blood pressure is restored to normal. This may be likened to the fact that you cannot fill a bath with water until you put in the bath plug and transfusion given before clamping the aorta is a waste of blood. When the patient's condition is stabilised the surgeon can get on with replacing the ruptured aorta with a Dacron graft. The operation is not difficult. The difficulty is to get co-operation to handle the case in sterile operating conditions in this way without routine theatre preparation (Fig. 91).

If the aneurysm is treated by an elective operation before rupture takes place it is exactly the same but the mortality is negligible, while the mortality of operative treatment of a ruptured aneurysm is about 40 % in the best hands.

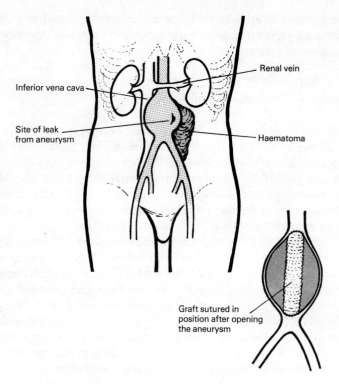

Inferior vena cava

Renal vein

Site of leak
from aneurysm

Haematoma

Graft sutured in
position after opening
the aneurysm

Fig 91   Abdominal aortic aneurysm

Postoperative Nursing Care and Observations

An elective operation does not usually merit postoperative treatment
in the intensive care unit but all patients who have had surgery for a
ruptured aneurysm will need intensive care. There are two aspects of
postoperative treatment. The first is concerned with maintenance of a
stable circulation with a blood pressure over 100 mmHg. A urinary
catheter is used to collect and measure urinary output as this is a
measure of renal function. The requirement for blood or other fluid
transfusion is assessed from the central venous pressure which is
measured with a catheter passed through a large vein and into the
superior vena cava. A low central venous pressure usually indicates
undertransfusion.

The second group of observations concern the technical aspects of
the operation. Any signs of local haemorrhage or excessive leak of
blood from the suction drains should be reported to the surgeon.

Thrombosis at the suture lines or embolus of thrombus from the aneurysm will result in ischaemic signs in the leg. The clinical appearance in the legs supported by pulse volume recordings are used to detect any deterioration in the circulation. This may be severe enough for the patient to be returned to the theatre for embolectomy.

Dissecting Aneurysm

This serious condition is usually caused by atherosclerosis. A split in the ascending aorta close to the heart allows the blood to run from the lumen into the wall of the aorta, where under the aortic blood pressure it dissects a layer in the wall of the aorta. While the main stream of aortic blood is intact a second stream runs in the wall and as dissection proceeds it compresses branches such as the subclavian artery causing obstruction to the subclavian artery flow. Eventually the second flow of blood may pass within the aortic wall as far as the abdominal aorta. Most cases die within a few hours, often as a result of haemorrhage from the dissection into the chest or abdomen.

There is very little hope of recovery but the surgical repair consists of replacing the ascending aorta with a Dacron graft. The coronary arteries have to be implanted into the graft and the operation is done under cardiothoracic bypass.

Diabetic Gangrene

In spite of many improvements in the treatment of diabetes it remains a very serious disease and the vascular complications cause a great deal of difficulty. Atherosclerosis develops early and is particularly widespread in diabetics. In this type of case, although reconstructive surgery may be considered for gangrene, the diffuse disease makes it less likely to be successful than in non-diabetic patients. In a second type of diabetic gangrene which occurs in young people, the arteries are normal and the foot pulses present yet there is infective, wet gangrene of the toes, often extending onto the foot. Because of the infective nature of the gangrene there is obvious putrefaction and a very offensive smell. In these cases the infection often extends to involve the bones of the toes and foot giving a characteristic appearance on an X-ray.

The treatment of diabetic gangrene is dependent on the type. If the gangrene is mainly due to atherosclerosis which has developed in a diabetic, the surgeon may try to do an operation of arterial reconstruction. But if the main arteries are normal and the foot pulses easily palpable the aim will be to give antibiotics to eradicate the infection and to remove any dead tissue including bone. Sometimes the foot infection is so extensive that a below knee amputation will be necessary but surgeons try to avoid this as the other foot may be affected by gangrene at a later date.

Diabetics are also liable to a complication called neuropathy because the peripheral nerves are affected and the limb becomes anaesthetic. This has one fortunate aspect because the patient does not suffer the pain which is felt so severely in ordinary atherosclerotic gangrene. However, another aspect is that the patient is very liable to develop a pressure necrosis. In bed, a patient usually lies with the foot externally rotated so that the outer side of the heel rests on the bed. As there is no sensation in the foot the patient does not know when pressure begins to cause ischaemia and does not move his foot as a patient with normal sensation would do. Various devices such as sheepskin rugs are used to reduce the effect of compression but there is no substitute for regular movement of the foot into different positions. The penalty of failure may be a large, deep, infected ulcer, which will take many weeks or months to heal.

Diabetics are prone to infection and special attention is paid to the feet to prevent injury which may be followed by a serious infection possibly leading to an amputation. Because the skin is anaesthetic a patient may not notice that a new pair of shoes is causing a blister or that he has received a foot injury while in a crowd. Careless nail cutting may result in a minor injury which becomes infected leading to disastrous consequences.

Buerger's Disease

The cause of Buerger's disease is unknown. It affects the feet of young men and there is no special racial predisposition. There is overactivity of the sympathetic nervous system manifested by sweating of the feet and arterial spasm causing pallor. Later the distal arteries of the foot become occluded leading to claudication in the foot (plantar claudication) and gangrene of the toes with normal foot pulses. The disease is much worse in cigarette smokers and can be arrested if the patient agrees to stop smoking.

If the disease is not arrested by stopping smoking the sympathetic overactivity can be corrected by doing a bilateral lumbar sympathectomy. Although this operation is quite easy there is a possibility of interfering with sex function which operates through the sympathetic nervous system and patients should always be warned of this possibility if lumbar sympathectomy is proposed on a young man. If gangrene of a toe is present it can be treated by amputation of the toe because the main arteries are normal. This should be compared with the old man with gangrene of the toe due to atherosclerosis. It is often difficult to explain to these patients that amputation of the toe will be followed by gangrene of the foot and that a thigh level amputation will be required. This is because in atherosclerosis the gangrene is caused by obstruction of the iliac or femoral arteries.

Raynaud's Disease

Raynaud's disease affects the hands of young women. A slightly different form of the disease is seen in premenopausal women. The appearance of the disease at these two ages strongly suggests that some abnormality of sex hormones is responsible but none has been identified and hormone treatment is not successful. The syndrome of Raynaud's disease is usually triggered by exposure to cold but in about one quarter of the cases the attack is brought on by some emotional stress.

The first phase of an acute attack of Raynaud's disease is an intense constriction of the small arteries in the fingers as a result of which they become white in colour. The spasm is gradually released and after a few minutes blood begins to pass through into the tissues which are starved of blood. All the oxygen is taken from the blood which results in the fingers turning blue in colour. As the spasm completely disappears blood floods into the fingers causing them to swell and become hot and red. In the most severe cases the recurrent attacks may result in terminal and painful gangrene of the finger tips. Mild cases are common and spontaneous improvement is likely. Severe cases are very rare.

A somewhat similar condition is called Raynaud's phenomenon. The attacks, which are similar to those of true Raynaud's disease, may be seen in young men with Buerger's disease and in patients of either sex with atherosclerosis. In cases which have been present for many years the skin of the fingers and hand may thicken – a condition called scleroderma.

If the patient complains that the symptoms are very severe the attacks can be prevented by doing an upper dorsal sympathectomy to cut off the sympathetic nerve supply to the small arteries of the fingers and so prevent vascular spasm.

Amputations

There are a number of conditions in which amputation is the only course open to the surgeon. One important indication for a major amputation is trauma, usually resulting from a road traffic accident. Young motor cyclists are particularly prone to serious leg injuries which cannot be repaired, making amputation the only possible treatment. At the other end of life there are still a number of amputations for arterial disease including gangrene resulting from atherosclerosis, diabetes or embolism. In some extensive malignant tumours the price of life may be a major amputation and some severe infections such as gas gangrene are treated by amputation.

In the leg the common sites for amputation include the midthigh amputation, Stokes-Gritti, and below knee amputation. The level of a mid thigh amputation is self evident. Stokes-Gritti is just above the knee joint and a below knee amputation is five to seven inches below the joint. The longer the stump the better the function.

In an older person, the high amputations give rise to severe disability, while a young person with a below knee amputation can lead an almost normal life. The surgeons will try to save as much leg as possible consistent with a good chance of primary healing.

The Amputation

The patient must be made as fit as possible by attention to cardiac function, anaemia, etc. before the operation. If there is frank gangrene the gangrenous part should be wrapped in a plastic bag before the patient goes to the theatre so that this highly infected part is not exposed in the theatre. The bag is not removed until the amputated leg leaves the theatre suite. Stumps are usually bandaged at the end of the operation. Some surgeons prefer to use Elastoplast as a bandage is very inclined to fall off an amputation stump. Suction drains are left in the wound and are removed after a few days when serous drainage has stopped.

There can be few cases in which so many departments of the hospital are involved with the postoperative care as with an amputation, particularly when it is done for senile gangrene.

Physiotherapy

The physiotherapist attends the patient before the amputation and begins the exercises which are so vital after the amputation and which are designed to prevent deformity and contracture of the joints and to preserve and improve the function in the muscles of the stump which remain. The modern operation is called a myoplastic amputation and this simply means that the muscles are cut longer than the bone so that they can be sutured over the bone end. This fixation results in better muscle function.

It is essential to get the patient out of bed and onto some form of artificial limb as soon as possible. The first aid to walking is the pneumatic limb, which can usually be fitted about the fifth to seventh day. This is simply a cylindrical shaped bag contained in a frame which is pumped up with the stump inside the bag so that it takes exactly the shape of the stump and evenly distributes the weight. The patient walks on a wooden rocker in the position of the shoe. Using this he is usually able to take a few steps with the aid of a Zimmer walking frame or with crutches (Fig. 92). Physiotherapy departments and some vascular wards are equipped with parallel bars so that the patient can walk on the pneumatic limb while taking the weight and steadying himself with his hands on the bars.

Physiotherapy in bed is designed to prevent joint contractures and to prevent muscle wasting. In thigh amputations a flexi n deformity at the hip can easily develop because while the patient is sitting the hip is acutely flexed and hip extension exercises are particularly important.

Social Services and Occupation Therapy Departments

After a successful amputation the patient will eventually be well enough to leave the hospital and hopefully return to his home and family. It may be that an elderly patient will not get on well with walking with an artificial limb and that he will be to some extent chairbound and will need a wheel chair to get about even at home. This is especially so after a bilateral amputation which may be necessary in elderly arteriosclerotics. The social service's workers visit the patient's home before he is discharged to ensure that it is possible for him to return in reasonable safety. If there are steps in the house it may be necessary for them to be converted to a ramp which can be used by the patient in a wheelchair. Hand holds in the toilet and alongside the bath are always necessary so that the patient can use his

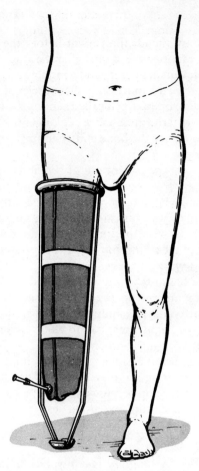

Fig 92   Pneumatic limb

hands to pull himself up from the bath or toilet. Even in the kitchen a few well placed hand holds may enable a patient to work and cook in the kitchen so retaining some degree of independence. When it seems time for an elderly amputee to return home it is better to send him for a trial weekend than to discharge him from the hospital. Only when he is able to show that he can get on at home is he finally discharged.

Limb Fitting Services

While the patient is in hospital an appointment is made for him to attend the limb fitting centre where he will be measured for an artificial limb. It takes about three months for a limb to reach its final size. Following the amputation there is swelling in the stump and it is necessary to wait for this to subside before the final limb is fitted. The patient is initially fitted with a pylon which is a temporary limb with a rocker foot like the pneumatic limb, and taking weight on the ischial tuberosity which is a bone in the buttock. As soon as this limb is available the patient is taught to walk at the limb fitting centre and with help from the physiotherapy department.

The final limb fits the stump snugly and is called a total weight bearing limb because it spreads the weight load over the whole stump. The modern limb does not have any straps to fit it to the patient. It is fitted with a matching shoe instead of a rocker and there is a locking device for the knee which is locked for walking but unlocked when the patient sits so that the knee can be flexed.

Psychological Support

Many patients dread the disability which will follow a major amputation and every possible support and encouragement is given. One of the best forms of encouragement is to introduce a patient who has successfully overcome the disability of a major amputation.

28

Veins

Anatomy and Physiology of the Leg Veins

Two systems of veins return blood from the leg towards the heart. The superficial veins are based on the long and short saphenous veins. The long saphenous vein can often be seen in front of the bone inside the ankle (the medial malleolus). From this point it takes a virtually straight course up the inner side of the leg to the groin. Just below the groin it dips through the deep fascia to join the femoral vein. Throughout its length the long saphenous vein receives tributaries carrying blood from the superficial tissues. The short saphenous vein runs behind the lateral malleolus and then up the middle of the back of the calf of the leg. Behind the knee it joins the popliteal vein.

The deep veins accompany the main arteries of the leg. Below the knee there are three arteries called the posterior tibial, anterial tibial and peroneal. At this level the deep veins are represented by two or three small veins rather than a single one. Just below the knee these veins all join to form the popliteal vein. This is a large vein which is continuous with the femoral vein in the thigh and the iliac vein in the pelvis. At about the level of the umbilicus the iliac veins from the two sides join to form the inferior vena cava.

The return of blood from the feet to the heart presents some difficulty in the upright posture of man. It is to some extent effected by the pressure from behind, which is the arterial pressure through the capillaries. All the veins are provided with numerous valves which prevent the blood from flowing back down the leg. The deep veins are surrounded by the muscles of the leg and are squeezed when the muscles contract in walking. The valves prevent reflux of blood when the vein is compressed so that it is propelled forwards towards the heart against the effect of gravity.

The superficial and deep systems of veins are connected by a number of veins which are called communicating veins or perforaters. Each communicating vein is provided with a valve which ensures that blood can only flow from superficial to deep. There are several communicating veins in the lower third of the leg and the blood from this area normally drains through these veins to the deep veins (Fig. 93).

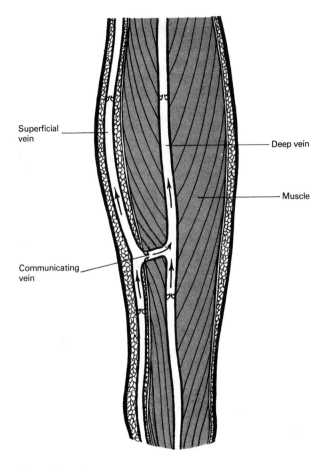

Fig 93   The calf muscle pump

Varicose Veins

Varicose veins are dilated and tortuous veins which are tributaries of the long or occasionally the short saphenous veins. As the varicose vein gets larger the valves are not large enough to control the reflux of blood and so the pressure in the vein increases and the varicose vein tends to get worse.

In most cases there is no obvious cause of varicose veins but compression of the veins in the pelvis impeding venous blood flow is an obvious possibility. The most common cause of obstruction is pregnancy and many pregnant women get varicose veins which regress after delivery of the baby. Varicose veins are more common in women than men because of the effect of pregnancy on the venous return.

Many women go to the doctor because of the unsightly appearance of varicose veins and ask for treatment for cosmetic reasons. In addition there are a number of complications.

1   Ankle oedema results from the increased pressure in the veins which is caused by the reduced venous return associated with incompetent valves. This increased tension in the leg accounts for some aching pain which is felt especially on standing.

2   Thrombophlebitis.   Varicose veins may suddenly, and for no obvious reason, undergo the complication of thrombophlebitis. The varicose vein becomes hard and very painful because of thrombosis and associated inflammation. The cause of the inflammation is uncertain but it is not bacterial and there is no place for antibiotic treatment. Patients with acute thrombophlebitis have difficulty in walking because of pain. The treatment is rest and the use of an anti-inflammatory drug. These drugs all have a tendency to cause acute ulcers of the stomach and duodenum and should only be given on a full stomach. External applications are often given but it is difficult to see how they can be of benefit.

3   Eczema.   Although eczema is a generalised disease it tends to be more severe in the legs with varicose veins and to be improved after treatment of the varices.

4   Venous ulcers are caused by incompetent perforators and are more commonly a complication of deep vein thrombosis. Many people have gross varicose veins without any sign of venous ulceration.

5   Bleeding from varicose veins can be very serious unless correct first aid is given. If a varicose vein is opened in an accident, blood pours out because of the incompetent valves in the vein above and people have been known to die of bleeding. The ill-advised and incorrect use of tourniquet may make matters worse. If the tourniquet is applied above venous and below arterial pressure the bleeding increases. Elevation of the leg with the patient lying flat on the ground stops the bleeding instantly.

Treatment of Varicose Veins

Injection Sclerotherapy

The principle of the modern technique is to inject an irritant substance into an empty vein. The vein is then compressed by bandaging with the object of securing adhesion of the two sides of the compressed vein and obliteration of the lumen. Injection of a full vein is likely to cause a local thrombosis in the varicose vein which will recanalise in a matter of months or a few years with recurrence of the varicose vein.

The needle is put into the full vein. This can be achieved with a venous tourniquet with the patient lying down or by asking the patient to stand. Five or six needles can be inserted before emptying the veins by removing the tourniquet or asking the patient to lie down. An injection of 1 ml of sodium tetradecylsulphate (STD) is given at each site. The co-operation of a nurse who understands the technique is essential as a bandage is applied to the leg with a foam pad over each injection to increase the compression at that point. The bandage is begun at the foot and extended up over each injection site as it is given. When the injection and elastic bandaging is completed an elastic stocking is put on. This external compression is kept on night and day for six weeks. The treatment is uncomfortable in the temperate English climate but in hot countries it is unacceptable to most patients.

There is always a risk that a local thrombosis will occur and that it will spread into the deep veins of the leg. To make this complication unlikely patients are told to walk at least two miles daily to keep a good flow of blood in the deep veins. In spite of this precaution there have been cases of deep vein thrombosis and pulmonary embolism following injection sclerotherapy and a few deaths have been recorded.

Patients should stop taking the contraceptive pill during sclerotherapy because of the known complication of thrombosis in patients using this form of contraception.

The main advantage of sclerotherapy is that it can be done in the outpatient department, which is more acceptable to the patient than admission to a hospital bed and is also cheaper.

Surgical Treatment

1   **Stripping.**   The standard operation in use for varicose veins is removal of the whole of the long saphenous vein by a technique called

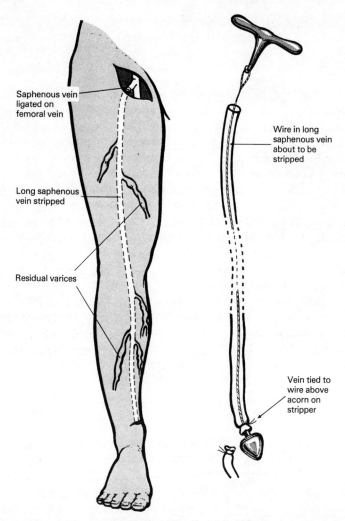

Fig 94 Operation for stripping long saphenous vein

stripping. In recent years cardiovascular surgeons have used the long saphenous vein for coronary artery and for femoral artery grafting so that it should not be removed unless it is grossly dilated.

In the stripping operation a wire is passed into the long saphenous vein at the ankle and passed proximally until it reaches the groin where it is passed out through the divided long saphenous vein. The vein is tied above an acorn at the ankle and the stripper pulled until it emerges with the whole long saphenous vein at the groin. In stripping the vein all its tributaries are torn off and the open ends bleed into the tissues.

Following the operation an elastic bandage is applied to the leg to compress the veins and to control bleeding into the tissues.

2 Sapheno-Femoral Ligation. This is an important part of most operations for varicose veins because the valve at the sapheno-femoral junction is often incompetent. The operation is done through a small incision at the top of the thigh and the saphenous vein ligated and divided just below the point at which it enters the femoral vein.

3 Multiple Excisions. The actual varices are best removed as they tend to persist even after stripping or ligation of the sapheno-femoral junction. The varices must be marked with ink before the operation as they cannot be seen when the patient is lying down and the veins are empty. The varices can be removed through tiny incisions which do not need sutures but can be closed with micropore tape. As each individual varix is teased out without ligation there is some bleeding from the ends and this is controlled with an elastic support. It is more comfortable for the patient if a tubinette (Seton) stocking is put on the leg which is then bandaged with Lestroflex. This support is removed after one week and replaced by a support of tubigrip (Seton) for a further week.

Postoperative Care of Varicose Vein Operation

1   If a sapheno-femoral ligation has been performed the wound should be inspected at intervals after the operation as the ligature sometimes slips off the saphenous vein and bleeding from the femoral vein causes a large haematoma in the groin. If this happens the surgeon should be informed. A large haematoma should be treated by exploration and ligature of the bleeding vein.

2   The elastic support which is put on to control bleeding may be applied too tightly. This is a dangerous situation as the effect may be like a tourniquet. If the patient complains that the bandage is painful and too tight it should usually be removed and reapplied. Tingling or anasthaesia in the foot are signs of ischaemia and the bandage should be removed at once.

If the leg is correctly bandaged the foot should remain a normal pink colour and any blue discolouration should be reported.

The foot of the bed is raised on blocks after any varicose vein operation to reduce swelling.

3   Unless there are social reasons to the contrary the patient is discharged on the day following the operation with instructions to keep active and walking. Standing should be avoided and if the patient is sitting the feet are elevated. One rare complication is spread of thrombosis from superficial to deep veins with risk of pulmonary embolus and this is made less likely by early mobility.

4   The patient is seen in the outpatient department on the seventh day when the sutures are removed from the groin wound.

Thromboembolism

Vein Thrombosis and Pulmonary Embolism

Thrombosis of veins in the leg or pelvis may occur without warning or apparent cause. Sitting in a car or aeroplane for many hours with the knee flexed partially obstructs the venous flow of blood and may cause the veins to thrombose. More commonly deep vein thrombosis is seen in patients who are in bed in medical wards or following operations. Such a thrombus inside a vein is not adherent to the wall of the vein when it first forms and it may not completely obstruct the lumen so that the thrombus hangs loosely in the stream of blood. This is a dangerous situation as a part of it may break off and be carried in the blood stream. It will pass up through the inferior vena cava to enter the right atrium of the heart. The thrombus then passes through the tricuspid valve to the right ventricle and then leaves the heart through the pulmonary artery. A large embolus will be unable to pass any further and will almost completely occlude the pulmonary artery. A smaller thrombus will pass through the main pulmonary artery into one of the lungs to be arrested in a branch of the pulmonary artery. This is called pulmonary embolism. If the embolus completely plugs the pulmonary artery and stops the circulation the patient complains of sudden severe central chest pain and may die in a few minutes. Embolism of a branch of the pulmonary artery also causes sudden chest pain but although there may be some dyspnoea recovery is usual. A small segment of lung is deprived of its blood supply and undergoes a pathological condition called infarction. After a few days the patient may notice blood in the sputum and complain of pain on breathing. This is called pleuritic pain and is caused by roughening of the pleura covering the infarcted lung. An infarcted segment of lung may be expected to revascularise and return to normal.

Site of Vein Thrombosis

1 Iliac Vein Thrombosis. Thrombosis of the iliac veins usually occurs in pregnancy or childbirth or following operation in the pelvis. As the complete venous return from the leg is obstructed the whole leg becomes swollen and the condition is sometimes called a white leg. There is a risk of pulmonary embolism but eventually the iliac vein is likely to recanalise. The leg may remain a little swollen but there is no risk of leg ulceration.

2 Calf Vein and Femoropopliteal Vein Thrombosis. Postoperative vein thrombosis usually begins in small tributaries in the calf muscles and spreads into the main veins of the leg and to the popliteal and femoral veins.

At this stage the patient complains of pain or stiffness in the calf and there is tenderness on pressure in the calf muscle. There is usually a low fever. Sometimes the leg is a little swollen and it may be warmer than its fellow. The superficial veins may appear a little distended. However, it must be emphasised that the clinical evidence of a deep vein thrombosis is not always obvious and the first sign may be a pulmonary embolus.

Following recovery the patient may be left with a condition of chronic venous insufficiency in the leg.

Diagnostic aids such as venography are not routinely used and treatment is based on the clinical diagnosis.

Prevention of Vein Thrombosis

A great deal of time has been spent trying to develop techniques which will prevent postoperative vein thrombosis and embolism.

1 External support with specially fitted elastic stockings is almost routinely used in America but is not widely used in Great Britain because there is insufficient data to justify the great expense involved in fitting every theatre patient with elastic stockings. The theoretical advantage is that bandaging compresses the superficial veins so directing the blood flow to the deep veins. It is supposed that this will increase the flow rate and make thrombosis less likely.

2 Anticoagulants. Normal doses of anticoagulants were used for many years in patients thought likely to get a deep vein thrombosis. A high incidence of postoperative haemorrhage made this technique unpopular. More recently a regime of low dose heparin has been used in some centres but it must be said that it is not widely used. In this technique 5000 units of heparin are given two hours before the operation and then eight hourly for seven days.

3   Elevation of the foot of the bed encourages venous return and may be helpful in preventing leg vein thrombosis.

4   Measures taken during surgery.   In some hospitals much reliance is placed on putting a pillow under the heels to take pressure off the calf. There is an electrical device to cause regular contractions of the calf muscle during the operation and an appliance which fits round the leg and contracts regularly in an attempt to mimic the action of the calf pump. All these techniques have been popular at times but none has received universal approval.

Treatment of Established Deep Vein Thrombosis and Pulmonary Embolism

1   Bed Rest

Once a deep vein thrombosis has been diagnosed the patient is at risk of a pulmonary embolus. Rest in bed reduces the risk of detachment of the thrombus through contractions of the calf muscle. The leg is often bandaged and the foot of the bed elevated. These two measures are designed to increase the flow of blood in the deep veins. The period of time that a patient is kept in bed is variable but the object is to keep the leg at rest until the thrombus is adherent to the wall of the vein so that the patient is no longer at risk of a pulmonary embolus.

2   Anticoagulants

These are routinely used in cases of deep vein thrombosis. Anticoagulants do not dissolve thrombus but they stop its propagation and probably reduce the incidence of embolism.

Anticoagulation is begun with heparin because it is effective immediately after an intravenous injection. Heparin is rapidly destroyed in the body and to keep up the level of anticoagulant in the blood it is given intravenously with a clockwork pump which drives a syringe and injects the heparin at a constant speed (Fig. 95). The

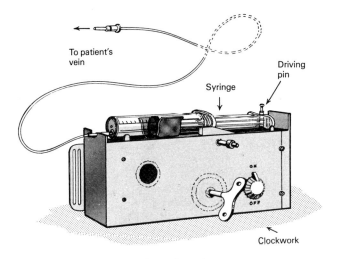

Fig 95 Constant infusion pump for IV heparin

usual regime is to give 5000 units intravenously as a bolus and then to give the 20 000 units every 12 hours. If heparinisation is to be continued for more than three days the effect on clotting has to be measured every day. This is done by estimating the plasma clotting time (PCT). The patient's plasma is tested against normal plasma by adding a substance called thrombin to each. It will cause rapid clotting of normal plasma but clotting will be delayed in the patient's plasma. For safe anticoagulation the PCT should be kept between two and three times normal.

It is generally considered that anticoagulant treatment should be continued for about three months. Warfarin is used for long anticoagulation. This drug is convenient for outpatients because it is given by mouth as a tablet. It cannot be used as the initial treatment because it does not cause effective anticoagulation for about two or three days. Warfarin and heparin are sometimes given together and the heparin stopped when the Warfarin effect is established. A daily maintenance dose of 5 – 10 mg is usual but this needs to be checked by doing a blood prothrombin time.

Chronic Venous Insufficiency in the Leg

Following a deep vein thrombosis in the leg there is partial or complete recanalisation of the thrombosed veins after a period of some months. However, there is usually some residual thrombus which partially obstructs the venous return and the valves which have been damaged by the thrombosis become incompetent. As a result the return of blood through the leg veins is slower than normal. In addition the valves in the perforating veins are damaged and incompetent so that on walking blood flows out through the communicating veins causing a rise in the pressure in the superficial veins and capillaries. The capillary circulation is slowed and the skin and fat become ischaemic. This results in an oedematous leg and often a chronic venous ulcer which is very resistant to treatment (Fig. 96).

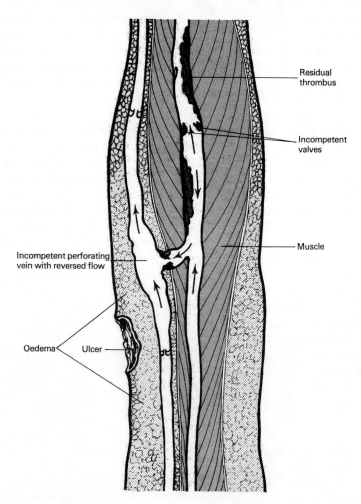

Fig 96 Abnormal venous return in chronic venous insufficiency

Treatment

Conservative treatment aims to heal the ulcer by restoring the venous circulation to normal. The best way to achieve this is by putting the patient to bed with the feet elevated so that the venous return from the leg is increased. This is often done to get an ulcer healed but it is likely to recur when the patient gets up again. Local dressings to a venous ulcer are not very critical but if the ulcer is infected it can be dressed with Eusol to encourage the separation of slough.

If the patient does not wish to spend some weeks in bed he may be treated by bandaging. The object of bandaging is to compress the openings of the perforating veins and prevent the flow of blood through them to the superficial veins. One popular support bandage is made of paste which sets to a firm consistency when exposed to air. The bandage is kept in an airtight plastic bag and used to bandage the leg from the toes to below the knee. It is changed at weekly visits to the clinic.

Any patient with chronic venous insufficiency needs to adapt his or her life in order to live in reasonable comfort without too much risk of recurrent venous ulceration. This particularly means avoiding standing still. Whenever possible the patient should sit and when sitting she should put her feet up on a support. A support bandage or elastic stocking is likely to be needed for life.

Surgical treatment is not very often used because results are not completely successful. The operation is to identify and ligate the perforating veins. The reason for a partially successful result is that the deep veins are still left with incompetent valves and poor function and only the incompetent perforators are dealt with by the operation. If an incision is made down the back of the calf the sutures should not be removed for at least ten days.

29

The Lymphatic System

Fluid passes out of the capillary blood vessels into the extracellular fluid of the body. About 65 % of the body water is inside the cells and is called the intracellular fluid and about 25 % is extracellular. This water contains electrolytes and protein and is the vehicle through which nutrients and oxygen pass from the capillary blood vessels to the cells. Water containing waste products and carbon dioxide from the cells is absorbed back into the capillaries. However, some water and protein is not reabsorbed. Indeed the protein cannot get back into the capillaries and this extra fluid and protein is absorbed into a network of tiny tubes called lymphatics. Bacteria causing an infection may also find their way into the lymph vessels. This network of fine tubes collects into larger tubes which have valves just like veins to encourage the flow of lymph inside the vessels. Lymph passes through lymph nodes which are spaced along the route. The nodes contain antibody-producing cells called lymphocytes and bacteria are often held up and destroyed in the lymph nodes. About five lymph vessels run up the leg and into the body taking a route alongside the main blood vessels. In the upper part of the abdomen all the lymph trunks join to form a larger sac called the cisterna magna and a large tube called the thoracic duct carries the lymph through the back of the chest. Finally the thoracic duct enters the neck and joins the left subclavian vein so returning the fluid and protein to the blood stream. A similar duct on the right side drains lymph from the right arm and right side of the head back into the blood stream (Fig. 97).

The lymphatic system serves a second important function. Fat which is digested in the intestine cannot be absorbed directly into the blood capillaries like the products of digestion of sugars and protein. Fat is absorbed into tiny lymph vessels in the intestine which empty into the cisterna magna in the abdomen. The fat particles pass through the thoracic duct and reach the blood stream where the thoracic duct enters the subclavian vein.

Oedema

Oedema is the retention of an excess of fluid in the extracellular space. There are two main causes:

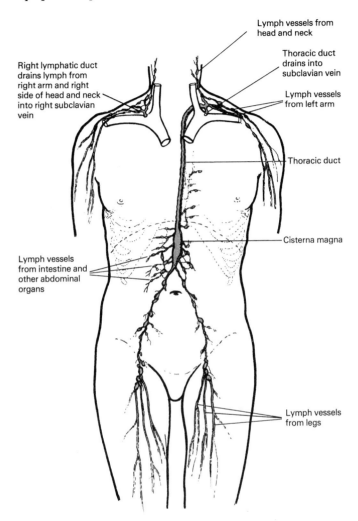

Lymph vessels from head and neck

Thoracic duct drains into subclavian vein

Right lymphatic duct drains lymph from right arm and right side of head and neck into right subclavian vein

Lymph vessels from left arm

Thoracic duct

Cisterna magna

Lymph vessels from intestine and other abdominal organs

Lymph vessels from legs

Fig 97 Anatomy of the lymphatic system

1   Venous Oedema

If there is any obstruction to the flow of blood in the veins the rise of pressure in the veins and consequently in the capillaries hinders the absorption of fluid from the extracellular fluid into the capillaries. Two common causes of venous oedema are cardiac failure and thrombosis of the veins in the leg or pelvis.

2   *Lymphatic Oedema*

This results if there is interference with the normal drainage of water
and protein through the lymphatics. Even if the veins are normal
oedema will result. There are several causes of lymphoedema. One is
a congenital condition in which the lymph vessels of the leg are
abnormal. The most common abnormality is that only one or two
hypoplastic vessels are present instead of the normal five. This is
inadequate and fluid collects in the foot and leg. This condition is
called lymphoedema praecox.

Lymphatic oedema also results from disease or surgical operations.
A massive involvement of the lymphatic nodes in the groin with
secondary deposits of cancer will prevent lymphatic flow and cause
oedema. Another common cause is seen in breast cancer. This may
result from too radical excision of the axillary nodes in the operation
of mastectomy or it may follow a combination of surgery and
radiotherapy when the combined effect may cause gross oedema of
the arm and hand.

Investigation and Treatment of Oedema

Lymph vessels can be seen by giving an injection of Patent Blue Dye
into the foot. The fine network of vessels is outlined in blue and soon
after a larger lymph vessel in the dorsum of the foot is seen. This can
be cannulated using a small incision under local anaesthetic and radio-
opaque dye injected to show the lymphatic vessels of the leg. In
addition to the study of oedema, lymphangiography can be used to
visualise lymph nodes in the pelvis and abdomen. In cases of cancer of
the uterus and in lymphomas this study can be used to identify nodes
which are involved and to plan treatment on the basis of the
information provided.

Lymphoedema has been extensively studied and a great deal is now
known about it. Unfortunately there is still no satisfactory surgical
treatment.

30

Portal Hypertension

Liver Blood Supply (Fig. 98).

The liver receives blood from two sources. One is the hepatic artery which brings oxygenated arterial blood from the aorta. This contributes 20 % of the blood which flows through the liver. The second source of blood is the portal vein which contributes 80 % of the liver blood flow. The portal vein receives blood from the spleen through the splenic vein and from the intestines through the superior mesenteric vein. The mesenteric vein carries the products of digestion of carbohydrates and proteins which are absorbed into the blood in the wall of the small intestine.

These two sources of blood are mixed in the capillaries in the liver. The arterial blood is a source of oxygen and food for the liver cells. The products of digestion contained in the portal blood are submitted to a variety of complicated biochemical changes in the liver cells. Finally the blood passes from the liver in three or four large veins called the hepatic veins which drain into the inferior vena cava.

Portal Hypertension

The normal pressure in the portal vein is about 20 cm of water and portal hypertension is present if the pressure is above this level. Portal hypertension is caused by an obstruction to the passage of blood from the portal vein to the inferior vena cava. Three types are described:

1 Pre-hepatic Obstruction

This means that the obstruction is in the portal vein itself and the only common cause is thrombosis of the portal vein. This may occur as a complication of infection at the umbilicus in infancy and is a cause of portal hypertension in children. Portal vein thrombosis also occurs in patients with cirrhosis of the liver.

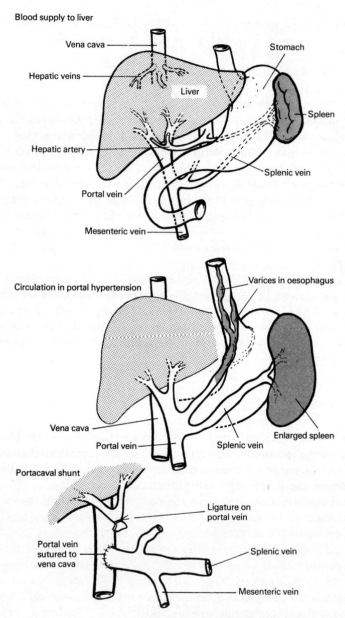

Fig 98   Normal blood supply to liver and portacaval shunt

2   Post Hepatic Obstruction

This is caused by thrombosis of the hepatic veins. This is a rare cause.

3   Hepatic Obstruction

Intrahepatic obstruction is by far the most common cause of portal hypertension. In many parts of the world, including the Middle East, it is caused by infection with a parasite called *Schistosomiasis*. The parasite lives in water and enters the skin of the feet. The adult worm matures and lives in branches of the portal vein where it causes an inflammatory reaction which results in thrombosis. The eggs from the adult worm spread in the blood steam to infect the bladder and rectum where they cause urinary or rectal symptoms. Thrombosis of the portal vein causes portal hypertension. The disease is called bilharzia and causes many deaths in the Middle East, particularly in Egypt.

In Europe, intrahepatic portal hypertension is usually caused by a disease called cirrhosis in which there is disorganisation of the normal microscoptic anatomy of the liver by fibrosis which obstructs the passage of blood through branches of the portal vein. The most common cause of cirrhosis with portal hypertension is an excessive intake of alcohol.

Effects of Portal Hypertension

The body responds to high pressure in the portal vein by developing alternative venous channels through which the portal blood can reach the vena cava without passing through the liver. These channels are between the portal vein or its tributaries and systemic veins which drain into the vena cava. There are many sites in the abdomen where these alternative channels, called shunts, can develop and they are generally beneficial because they contribute to lowering the portal blood pressure. However, one site of the natural venous shunt is through veins which are in the wall of the stomach and oesophagus. When these dilate they bulge like varicose veins into the lumen of the stomach and oesophagus and they may rupture causing catastrophic haemorrhage into the oesophagus (Fig. 98).

The raised pressure in the portal vein and the splenic vein causes enlargement of the spleen (splenomegaly).

The effects of cirrhosis are also seen in many cases of portal hypertension. The liver function may be well compensated but more severe cases show characteristic signs.

Peripheral oedema and ascites are caused by hypoalbuminuria (low blood albumin). This results from impaired liver function because the liver is the sole source of blood albumin. In severe cases there are signs of interference with brain function called portasystemic encephalopathy (PSE) or hepatic encephalopathy. There is a flapping tremor of the hands and the patient may become confused before lapsing into hepatic coma. There is some debate about the cause of these symptoms but ammonia has been incriminated. Ammonia is normally present in portal blood but destroyed in the liver. If it passes directly into the systemic blood without passing through the liver it reaches the brain and causes the symptoms of portasystemic encephalopathy. An excessive intake of protein, which is the source of ammonia, can exacerbate the symptoms and after a haemorrhage from oesophageal varices, portasystemic encephalopathy may develop because of the absorption of the protein in the blood passing through the intestine.

Investigation and Management of a Case of Portal Hypertension

If the patient is admitted as an emergency with haematemesis thought to be caused by ruptured oesophageal varices the first measures are directed to saving him from death, from loss of blood and hypovolaemic shock. All the vital functions are monitored. The pulse rate and blood pressure are measured and charted at 15 minute intervals in the early management. A urinary catheter is passed to measure the urinary output and the central venous pressure is monitored. A separate venous line is inserted for transfusion of blood in a quantity needed to combat the hypovolaemic shock.

Before contemplating special treatment for the varices it is necessary to confirm the diagnosis by endoscopy. In about 30% of patients with known portal hypertension the bleeding will be found to originate in a gastric or duodenal ulcer.

If the origin of the bleeding is shown to be oesophageal varices the conservative measure of blood transfusion is continued but some additional measures may be taken.

Intravenous pitressin is given because it has a specific action of reducing the flow of blood in the portal system and so lowering the

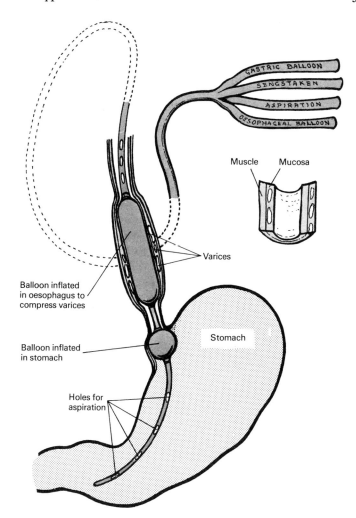

Fig 99 Sengstaken tube

portal pressure. If bleeding continues a Sengstaken balloon is inflated in the oesophagus (Fig. 99). The balloon in the stomach is inflated after passing the tube and it is then pulled out as far as possible so that the balloon is at the cardia. The oesophageal balloon is then inflated to compress the oesophageal varices and to control bleeding. At this stage the oesophagus is completely obstructed so that there is no possibility of oral feeding and the patient is hydrated and, if necessary, nourished by the intravenous route. An additional problem which results from oesophageal obstruction is that swallowed saliva will collect in the oesophagus and may reflux into the trachea causing inhalation pneumonitis and collapse. The modern modified Sengstaken tube has a fourth channel for aspiration of the oesophagus above the balloon. If this channel is absent or blocked it is an essential part of the nursing management to aspirate the pharynx with a sucker to prevent inhalation.

When the patient's condition is stable the Sengstaken tube is removed. Unfortunately this is often followed by recurrent bleeding so that some additional measure is required for longer term control.

The techniques at present under trial are directed at the oesophageal varices. In some centres they are treated by resection of the oesophagus and re-anastomosis. Complete division of the oesophagus also divides the varices and isolates the varices in the oesophagus from the high pressure in the portal vein. The operation is done through an incision in the abdomen. The stomach is opened and the staple gun described in Chapter 18 is used for the operation.

Although oesophageal bleeding can be arrested by this operation an even easier technique is to inject the varices in the same way as varicose veins in the leg. Although injection treatment was described in 1955 the enthusiasm for shunt operations blinded surgeons to the success of the technique which has only become popular in recent years. The injection is done using a rigid endoscope and the postoperative care depends on the type of anaesthetic used. If a local anaesthetic and sedation is used the patient must not have any oral fluid for four hours because when the pharynx is anaesthetised fluid may pass into the trachea as easily as into the oesophagus.

Shunts which are described later have little or no place in the treatment of acute bleeding from varices.

In many other cases the patient with cirrhosis is admitted with a history of recurrent haematemesis for elective treatment.

For many years these patients were treated by a variety of shunts. In the most popular the portal vein was transected and sutured into the vena cava, so diverting the portal blood from its normal route into the low pressure vena cava (Fig. 98). This operation was quite successful in stopping recurrent bleeding but a large number developed hepatic encephalopathy because of the passage of portal blood directly to the vena cava and so to the brain without first passing through the liver where the toxic substances such as ammonia were chemically changed.

There is at present a strong trend towards treating oesophageal varices with injection sclerotherapy. As with varicose veins in the leg there is a tendency for the varices to recur but they can be treated again if this happens.

Cirrhosis is a disease which is treated medically and the complication of portal hypertension is moving into the field of treatment by the endoscopist. At the present time the place of surgical treatment is very limited and will possibly disappear altogether.

31

Tissue and Organ Transplantation

The idea that diseased tissue or organs might be replaced is very old but technical and ethical problems have been very considerable.

There are two main types of graft:

1   The **autograft** which is a graft of tissue from one part of a patient to another part of the same patient. There are, of course, no ethical problems. Nor are there any problems of compatability of the graft as it is not moved to a different host. Examples of autografts are the split skin graft and the long saphenous vein graft which may be transplanted to replace an artery which is occluded.

2   The **allograft** (previously called a homograft) is taken from a donor of the same species, i.e. from one human being who is the donor to another who is the recipient. The allograft has formidable ethical and technical problems but the advantage to the recipient of a new organ such as a kidney (Fig. 100) may be nothing short of saving and prolonging life.

There are two other definitions which are useful. An **isograft** is one between identical twins who will possess identical genetic

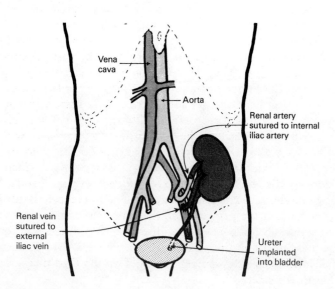

Fig 100   Kidney transplant

structure. There are no rejection problems in such a graft. A **xenograft** (previously called a heterograft) is one which is taken from an animal of a different species, e.g. a monkey kidney might be used to replace a human kidney. Although the supply of grafts would be unlimited the protein structure is so different that this type of graft has no place at the present time although future research may make it possible.

Allografts – the Ethical Problem

One source of a kidney is a close relative who is prepared to sacrifice one kidney. Even this has problems of matching but they are much less than with an unrelated donor. This technique can only be used for organs which are paired and the heart and liver are not available for transplant from living donors. The second source of a graft is a cadaver. The problem with cadaver grafts is that they deteriorate very quickly, immediately that the heartbeat stops, and the graft should be taken while the heart is still beating. This has led to a modification of the definition of death which has traditionally been defined as cessation of the heartbeat and breathing. With the development of intensive care units it has been possible to sustain life with life support systems so that, for example, breathing is dependent on the working of a machine. If it can be shown that the brain is dead and that there is no hope of recovery a decision to switch off the respirator has, eventually, to be made. This decision is not in any way connected with the possibility of donation of organs. It has lead to a new definition of death, brain death, in which the part of the brain called the brain stem is dead. The definition of brain death has been the subject of much research and precise criteria are now considered before making a diagnosis. Of course the public anxiety is that if a mistake is made a patient who might fully recover will have his life terminated by switching off the respirator. The diagnosis of brain stem death has to be made by two independent doctors who are not members of a transplant team. The main observations which are made concern the absence of certain reflexes which are dependent on a living brain stem. The pupils are large and do not react to light. The corneal reflex and the gag reflex in the throat are absent. Ice water injected slowly into the external auditory meatus does not result in any eye movement and respiration is absent when the respirator is switched off. These tests are repeated before the final diagnosis of brain death is made.

Many subjects are unsuitable as donors. Those with malignant

disease (except primary brain tumours), infections, advanced atherosclerosis and kidney disease are all unsuitable as donors. Many
potential donors are young people who have been involved in
accidents and have sustained severe head injuries at the time of the
accident. If a patient seems likely to be a potential donor extra blood
may be taken at the time of a necessary venopuncture for tissue
typing.

According to the Human Tissue Act of 1961 the person lawfully in
charge of the body is the only one who can authorise removal of
organs. If a patient dies in hospital this is the Health Authority until
such time as the next of kin, or in some cases the coroner, claims the
body.

The removal of organs for transplantation is discussed with the
next of kin. If the patient was carrying a signed donor card there is no
legal obligation to ask for the permission of relatives but it is regarded
as good practice to do so and indeed the whole question of dealing
with relatives must be conducted with the maximum of sensitivity as
they are already suffering from severe strain and distress.

Allografts – the Technical Problem

During the course of millions of years of evolution the body has
developed a variety of mechanisms to reject foreign protein. The
object has been to destroy and reject bacteria which invade the body
from time to time and which would lead to death if allowed to
multiply and spread. Unfortunately, the body is unable to distinguish
between the foreign protein of bacteria and the foreign protein of a
transplant and both are attacked in the same way. This is called the
immunological response and its success in eradicating infection is
matched by the problem of rejection which is one of the great
problems of an allograft.

Blood transfusion is the most common type of allograft. Its success
depends on the knowledge that there are four different blood groups
and a number of additional subgroups. With this knowledge blood of
the correct and compatible group is transfused. In addition blood cells
are constantly replaced from the bone marrow. The normal life of a
blood cell is about 100 days so that the problem of rejection is not
important except at the initial transfusion when a mis-matched
transfusion can be disastrous.

The same technique applied to tissue typing is much more
complicated. Foreign protein which enters the body is called an
antigen and it causes the production of a substance called antibody

which neutralises the antigen and causes it to be destroyed. These antigens can be detected on human white blood cells (leucocytes) and are called human leucocyte antigens (HLA). Unfortunately, many antigens are involved so that an exact match of the donor and recipient antigens is impossible and some degree of rejection is likely except in the case of a transplant between identical twins who have identical protein structure and identical antigens. The tissue data concerning possible recipients are kept on a computer at the United Kingdom Transplant Centre in Bristol and this holds data for all recipients waiting a kidney graft in Great Britain and much of Europe. Leucocytes from a possible donor are tissue typed and the information fed into the computer to try and identify a recipient who would give the best tissue match.

A second main problem is the time factor. When the heart stops the tissues are starved of oxygen and all tissues begin to deteriorate and eventually die. It is therefore preferable to harvest grafts from a subject who has been diagnosed as suffering from brain stem death but still has a beating heart.

When a graft is removed from the body it is perfused through the main artery with a special solution to remove blood and then stored at 4°C. The time in store is called the period of cold ischaemia and should not exceed 24 hours. During this time the graft and the recipient, who has already been identified from the computer, are both transferred to the same hospital. The period between cessation of the circulation to the graft and cooling it is called the period of warm ischaemia. This must be as short as possible because deterioration of ischaemic cells is rapid at body temperature.

Organs Available for Transplant

Transplants of cornea are used in patients with scars on the cornea causing blindness. These grafts have generally been more successful than other types of allograft because the lack of blood vessels in the cornea prevents the formation of antibody and subsequent rejection. When the cornea has blood vessels invading it the graft is subject to rejection like other allografts. The most commonly used organ allograft is the kidney transplant. Heart, liver and pancreas have been used as transplants but the problems are great and at present these grafts are still in the experimental stage. The expense is also enormous. There is a shortfall of about 50 % in available kidney grafts and for those successfully grafted with a cadaver allograft only about 30 % are still functioning five years later.

Following a transplant the patient is given drugs to suppress the immunological response which causes rejection. These are called immunosuppressive drugs. The most popular drugs have been azothioprine and corticosteroids. Recently the drug Cyclosporin A has shown promise. Corticosteroids have the disadvantage of causing an alteration in the facial appearance and in the longer term there is decalcification of the bones and possible fracture. The chemical immunosuppresive drugs make invasive infections more likely and there is also an increased incidence of cancer.

Appendix

After blood is collected for laboratory tests it is put into glass containers which are colour coded according to the chemical which they contain. Before collecting blood the correct container needed for the particular test is selected. (See table opposite).

Test	Volume	Container	Normal value in SI Units
Amylase	5 ml	White	50 – 300 units/l
Calcium	10 ml	Orange	2.4 – 2.8 mmol/l
Cholesterol	5 ml	White	3.6 – 7.8 mmol/l
ELECTROLYTES	10 ml	Orange	
Sodium			135 – 145 mmol/l
Potassium			3.5 – 5.5 mmol/l
Chloride			100 – 110 mmol/l
Bicarbonate			26 – 30 mmol/l
Urea	5 ml	Orange	2.3 – 6.5 mmol/l
LIVER FUNCTION	10 ml	White	
Bilirubin			2 – 17 μ mol/l
Alkaline phosphatase			5 – 35 units/l
Aspartate transaminase			Less than 50 units/l
Protein (total)			65 – 80 g/l
Full Blood Count and Haemoglobin	5 ml	Pink	
Acid phosphatase	10 ml	White	0 – 5 units/l
Prothrombin (BSR)	up to 2.5 ml mark	Mauve (container kept in refrigerator)	10 – 14 seconds

The mole (mol) is the SI unit of quantity. Its exact definition is complicated and it is convenient to consider the mole simply as a number. Concentrations are expressed as moles per litre (mol/l). The millimole (mmol) is 1000 times smaller and the micromole (μ mol) is one million times smaller than the mole.

Index